ERIC IS WINNING !!

ERIC IS WINNING !!

Beating a Terminal Illness with Nutrition, Avoiding Toxins and Common Sense

REVISED
EIGHT EDITION

ERIC EDNEY

To order additional copies of this book, contact:
Xlibris Corporation
1-888-795-4274
www.Xlibris.com
Orders@Xlibris.com
25941

Contents

Introduction 7

Preface 11

Chapter 1: The Bad News 13

Chapter 2: ALS Basics & My Program Basics 17

Chapter 3: Foundation For My Program 21

Chapter 4: Pre-established Beliefs 35

Chapter 5: Toxins – Possible Cause Of ALS
& Other Chronic Illnesses 43

Chapter 6 : The Beginning Of ALS–1990 Thru 1996 65

Chapter 7: Avoid All Toxins 75

Chapter 8: Detoxify The Body 105

Chapter 9: Diet & Dietary Supplements 123

Chapter 10: Starting A New Program 139

Chapter 11: Driving A Car 145

Chapter 12: My ALS Symptoms 147

Chapter 13: The ALS Comeback 155

Chapter 14: Doing It Over 165

Chapter 15: Motivation 171

Chapter 16: Summary 173

Updates 181

ALS Regimen Outline (Revised 12-1-05) 205

INTRODUCTION

by
Neal Rouzier, M.D.
Palm Springs, California

When I first read Eric Edney's account of how he halted the progression of ALS I was impressed that a layperson could have so much insight into health. At the same time I was disappointed that it was not a healthcare professional that was telling us what to do and what not to do. Although I sincerely commend Eric for his excellent commentary, I cannot help feeling disappointed in the obvious deficit in the way conventional medicine treats those with difficult diagnoses as well as age-related health problems. Despite the incredible wonder drugs and sophisticated technology to save lives, most medicine isn't practiced with an eye to longevity or optimal health. Instead, most conventional physicians remain occupied with prescribing drugs to treat established diseases as opposed to preventing them.

I am a conventional physician, yet there is no conventional treatment that helped Eric. I too am an alternative physician because that's all that has worked for Eric. One could also call it preventive medicine. The various treatments and regimens that Eric recommends are not specific for ALS or any other disease entity. He practices simple, basic preventive medicine, which should be practiced by all humans and taught by all physicians. Most simply, put back into the body those things that are missing. Take out those elements that are harmful, avoid anything toxic, eat the correct diet, take the correct supplements, exercise, love and respect one another. Unfortunately this simple solution is not found in any medical textbook.

Perhaps you would have had pity for Eric when he could not feed himself, hold a fishing pole or do one push up. That's the old Eric. Even though he still has the stigmata of ALS, the new Eric will out-fish you, do 20 push ups, 100 leg presses, and crush your hand in a handshake. If you could have seen him then and see him now, you would be impressed. He has managed to stop the progression of his disease as well as dramatically improve his residual function, which, up until now, has not been possible. He has successfully overcome that which no one else would think possible. And to give credit where credit is due, everything Eric does is not from my recommendation but through his own research and knowledge. Kudos to Eric!

The challenge for practitioners with a holistic/functional/integrative approach is to step back and look at the big picture: What are the ways to fine tune an aging body formed by bad habits, environmental factors, genetics, diet and laziness? To me Eric has been a teacher from whom I will learn and pass on to others. This global view of healthy aging or preventive medicine takes us far beyond conventional medicine and becomes a challenge for we physicians who have witnessed successes like Eric. The ravaging effects of chronic inflammation and toxins in the body will continue to wreak havoc and result in degenerative illness for millions in spite of simple therapies which can prevent this. It is my hope that this book will enlighten many so that they may not suffer the consequences of a degenerative illness. Don't just treat the disease; build up the body so it can put up a good fight.

As a physician I look for the learning opportunities in unforeseen detours of life. It may seem bizarre to look at a life-threatening disease as an opportunity for growth and learning, but that is exactly what has taken place here. ALS was an unplanned obstacle in the adventure of life for Eric. Imagine that a wise teacher has set up your life. Each obstacle was placed to teach you a needed lesson. This wise teacher provides these hurdles so that you and others may learn.

I have learned to value the lessons taught to me by the precious and fragile adventure of life. So has Eric. Now my greatest challenge is to evaluate patients from what I've learned from Eric before life takes them on an unplanned detour. This will make my medical practice distinctly satisfying. And for Eric, directing and helping others has made life more satisfying. That's why he wrote this book. Thank you, Eric.

And PS – Never stop learning.

Neal Rouzier, M.D.

PREFACE

You've heard the tale of David and Goliath? This is my David's (Eric's) story about how he has tamed that awful Goliath (ALS). It was back in 1996 when we received the fourth and final diagnosis of ALS. Eric told me then that he would beat this dreaded illness. I admired his Positive Mental Attitude, but I had my serious doubts and a million fears. In the last eight years, I have seen an amazing improvement in his physical condition. He is a remarkable man. Oh, there have been times I could have killed him, and I may still, but so far we have both survived. This is a story of his fourteen years with ALS. It includes his theories and his complete program with everything he did down to the last detail. This book should be interesting and informative to anyone in the healthcare business and certainly to anyone with a chronic illness such as ALS, Alzheimer's, MS, or other neurological ailment. This is a story of hope . . . . for Eric . . . . for me . . . . and for anyone who is fortunate enough to read his narrative.

Glenna Edney
Wife and caregiver for Eric these past fourteen years

CHAPTER I

THE BAD NEWS

It was a typical warm and sunny southern California morning in the fall of 1996 as we headed up the I-10 freeway from where we lived in Desert Hot Springs to the Loma Linda University Medical Center. My wife, Glenna, and I were both apprehensive about our appointment with the neurologist. The doctor had performed several tests on me in the previous months and we had arrived at Loma Linda that morning to learn the results. I had been diagnosed a few years earlier by a different doctor. However, since my previous doctor had only tested me for all 'treatable' illnesses, he did not give me a firm diagnosis at that time.

We parked our pickup truck and Glenna took my electric cart off the lift where we carry it on the back of the pickup. I can only walk a short distance with the aid of a walker, so I use an electric cart most of the time. A few minutes later we were in the doctor's office. The doctor told us that the results of one test had not come in yet, but he was almost certain that I had ALS or Amyotrophic Lateral Sclerosis a.k.a. Lou Gehrig's disease.

This was quite disturbing because most medical doctors will tell you ALS is a terminal illness and there is no known cure or treatment. They say you have from two to five years to live (from the date of diagnosis). Even though I had this ALS condition for five years prior to my visit to Loma Linda, I did not consider it to be terminal. I remained very hopeful. To suddenly call it ALS was more like saying you have inoperable cancer.

What was even more disturbing was the information booklet that the doctor gave me to take home and read. It said, in so many words, that you are going to die, and there are no exceptions. Go home and put your affairs in order. To say this was disturbing is putting it mildly. It was a shock! Since I was first diagnosed three years earlier, I figured this meant I wouldn't live more than another year, if that. The doctor's information booklet gave absolutely no hope-none-zip-zero! In fact, the doctor's booklet said specifically 'Don't even look for any treatment. There is none.'

Death from ALS could be a blessing in disguise when you consider the alternative. Living with ALS is a real nightmare. Here's what happens. First, the motor neuron brain cells begin to die. These are the brain cells that control your muscles and, therefore, all of your movement. Then, the muscles get weaker and eventually quit working. Of course, the muscles atrophy. This usually occurs in just one area at first, like an arm or a leg, but eventually leads to a shut down of your entire muscle system. The worst part is your brain remains active and unaffected. You wind up with a healthy brain in a dead body; perhaps the worst of all nightmares.

Later, I found out that this so-called specialist didn't really have all the facts. The truth is there are many long-term survivors with ALS: some 15 years, 20 years and more. Many of these are aided with a mechanical breathing apparatus and a feeding tube directly into the stomach. There are even some who have survived 20 years or more without any mechanical apparatus. As I look back, it is just as well that the doctor painted such a bleak picture for me, because it literally scared the hell out of me and really motivated me to do something. I went home from that visit to Loma Linda in the fall of '96 thinking I was going to die soon. However, it has been seven years and I am absolutely *no worse* in any area and actually have improvement in all areas.

Here's what happened next. I accepted this death sentence for a while, but after a couple of weeks I changed my mind. I decided there had to be a cure for ALS and I was going to find it. I'm sure there have been many people before me with this thought who failed. I don't want you to think that I absolutely knew that I could do it. However, I knew the only way to approach the problem was with a positive mental attitude. Sure, I knew it was a long shot, but I had to believe I could do it and I would not allow other negative thoughts to hang around. I told my wife in late 1996 that I would cure my ALS and I'm sure she did not believe me. However, I think by now I have convinced her.

You see, facing ALS was not the first time I thought that I was going to die.

In April of 1958, I was involved in a car accident. My former wife and I were stopped at a traffic light in our '57 Ford Ranchero pickup. A stolen car the police were chasing hit us from behind. A policeman said that the other car was traveling between 70 and 100 mph when they hit us. Our Ranchero was thrown into a traffic signal pole knocking it down. A bystander told me there was an explosion and a fireball that went about 30 feet in the air. Both doors were jammed and could not be opened. There was fire inside the Ranchero and I was being burned. I remember thinking I would most certainly die because no one would get us out in time. I thought how horrible the next few minutes would be! Then I suddenly changed my mind. I thought there had to be a way out. I thought of kicking out the windshield but decided the driver's door window would be much easier. I stood up on the seat and with my left foot I totally eliminated the window with one kick. Amazing what adrenaline will do. Next, I dove out the window headfirst and did a tuck-and-roll on the pavement. Fortunately, I had been a gymnast in high school. I had a horrible feeling about leaving my pregnant wife in the Ranchero, but I just had to get away from the burning flames. Being burned is extremely painful. I just had to get out of there even if it meant leaving her behind. After I dove out, I was on my feet in a matter of seconds. The only pedestrian within blocks approached me and asked if there was anyone else in the vehicle. I said yes. We rushed over and pulled my wife out through the window of the Ranchero and to safety. Fortunately, she was not burned. We both survived with only minor injuries. Our son, Rick, was born perfectly healthy about two weeks later.

The main message of this story is that you never want to quit even when things look pretty grim. In other words, don't give up! Additionally, you can't always rely on someone else to help you out of your predicament whatever it may be.

CHAPTER 2

ALS BASICS &
MY PROGRAM BASICS

Now that I have ALS, an untreatable and terminal disease, where did I get the idea that I could cure it? After all, I am not a medical doctor, I have had no medical training, and I am not a health practitioner of any sort. Actually, I think I know what gave me the idea. I have cured myself of psoriasis and arthritis when the medical doctors offered no effective treatment. The idea that I could cure myself of ALS came from my PMA (Positive Mental Attitude); I knew there had to be a way. I began by simply gathering all of the available information, putting it together, and applying some common sense. I should point out here that these ideas are not mine alone. There are many medical doctors including neurologists who follow the same thoughts about toxins. In other words, the theories put forth in this book are not mine alone. Let's review some of the information I have gathered. Here are a few facts about ALS and people with ALS:

ALS affects around 30,000 here in the United States. (It was 30,000 when I wrote this two years ago, but the latest figures are 35,000.) There are about 5,000 new patients or "People with ALS" (PALS) per year; that's about one in 50,000.

The average age at onset for ALS is 54.

Twice as many men get ALS as women.

Most PALS (People with ALS) are, or have been, very active physically.

A good majority of PALS are college graduates and/or very successful people.

It is estimated that only 40% of the U.S. population have amalgam dental fillings, while 90% of PALS have amalgam dental fillings (that is according to my own personal survey). Note: Amalgams contain mercury.

There are pocket areas of the population where ALS occurs far more frequently as on the island of Guam and with U.S. veterans of Desert Storm.

Some families have a far greater frequency of ALS than others do. They have a separate name for this. It is Familial ALS. It is still ALS anyway you slice it.

In a town called Plainfield, Vermont, there is an unusual cluster of ALS. Six people out of 1300 have ALS. Coincidentally, there was a salvage yard in the area where they burned tires by the carloads, no doubt putting out toxic fumes in the air.

Dairy farmers are four times more likely to get ALS.

All the above clusters or pockets of ALS would tend to indicate that there is something toxic in the environment in those areas.

ALS is not technically a disease. Rather, it is simply a condition of the body; a reaction to something unknown.

There is *no single test* by which one can diagnose ALS. The doctors test you for everything else possible. If that is all negative and you have ALS symptoms, then the conclusion is you have ALS.

Frequently the onset of ALS is preceded by a physical trauma.

Some of these facts would tend to indicate that the cause of ALS is in the environment; that is, the air we breathe, the water we drink, and the food we eat. We all know that there are toxins in the air, water and food. There is smog in the air, chlorine and fluoride in the water, and many different additives and preservatives in the food. Many of these are toxic. According to the US EPA, several thousand food additives are intentionally added to our food supply every year. The average American **eats 124** pounds of **food additives** a year. That is as much as my wife's total body weight. Additionally, over 2.5 billion pounds of pesticides and herbicides are dumped on our crop land, forests, lawns, and fields. If that isn't enough, we release over 4 billion pounds of chemicals into the ground and over 260 million pounds of chemicals into our lakes, rivers and oceans.

Here is what we know for sure. ALS and a number of other ailments including atherosclerosis, most forms of cancer, osteoporosis, multiple sclerosis, Alzheimer's disease, arthritis, and hypercholesterolemia are all much more common in the countries we refer to as Western civilization, and in fact only began occurring frequently in the last 200 years. Western civilization includes primarily the U.S. and a few European countries. The death rate from ALS has dramatically increased in these countries in the last twenty years. It, therefore, becomes obvious that Western countries are doing something to cause ALS and these other ailments. Additionally, we know that these same countries have been creating many more toxins in the environment and the exposure to toxins has been increasing rapidly in that same time period. Now, even a second-grader ought to be able to put those two facts together and draw a conclusion. The conclusion is (in case there are any first-graders reading this) that there is a high probability that one could be causing the other. Is it really hard to understand that our increased use of and exposure to toxins could be causing these ailments? Well, I don't think it is far-fetched at all.

Now let's look at the age of onset for ALS. The fact that the average age at onset is 54 would tend to indicate that we have been exposed to something for 20 or 30 years before it finally affects us. Could it be toxins?

Based on the idea that toxins could be the *cause*, I decided that the cure for ALS had to center on the cause. My plan was based on one simple belief; that a toxin or a combination of toxins causes ALS. I believe there is more than one toxin that can cause ALS. Further, the toxin that causes your ALS might be different from the toxin that causes mine. However, which toxin causes ALS is not that important at this point because there's only one thing to do anyway. You see, now that you already have ALS, the body is in a weakened condition. The only logical thing to do is to *avoid all toxins*, regardless of which one might have caused your problem. Since developing my plan in the fall of

1996, I have read articles and books written by medical doctors, some of whom are neurologists, which confirm my theory on toxins. There will be more detail on this later.

The plan involved **three steps:**

1. **Avoid exposure to any and all toxins.**
2. **Take all reasonable treatments to *remove* toxins from the body.**
3. **Provide the body with proper diet and dietary supplements.**

Additionally, I found a nutritionist to help me with my diet and dietary supplements. This I would wholeheartedly recommend to anyone seeking to follow a similar program.

Here is the basic idea. You want to give the body every opportunity to heal itself by making your body as *pristine* as possible. After all, the body heals itself; not the doctor. All you or any health practitioner can do is help. In the above three steps, you are doing everything possible to help your body. Incidentally, there are no known drugs that have any worthwhile affect on ALS. The only known drug that has a positive affect on ALS is Rilutek. At least that is the only drug approved by the FDA. The best it hopes to do is extend your life by a few months, and it only does that for a small percentage of people. Well, in my book, that is no solution and hardly worth mentioning. Additionally, Rilutek costs around $9,000 for one year of treatment in the U.S.

The above steps may sound simple enough, and they are; yet it is very upsetting to your lifestyle. That third step, proper diet, is a real 'doozy'. For the 40 years prior to this, I thought a day had to start with coffee, the evening had to include two or three beers, and it all ended with a bowl of ice cream about an hour after dinner. Well, as you might guess, all of that had to go, plus a lot more!

CHAPTER 3

FOUNDATION FOR MY PROGRAM

I could add a fourth step. However, it really isn't a step, but absolutely critical to your success. It is the *foundation* for a successful program to improve your health. You can't build a quality structure on a pile of sand. You must have a solid foundation.

Let me throw in a little philosophy before we start with the foundation.

> *A LITTLE ADVERSITY CAN MAKE AN EVENT MORE*
> *FUN!*
> *OVERCOMING GREAT ADVERSITY CAN BE A REAL*
> *ACHIEVEMENT!*

Overcoming ALS can be the challenge of a lifetime and your greatest accomplishment.

Now let's discuss the foundation for this accomplishment:

> *YOU MUST BELIEVE.*

That is, you must believe in what you're doing and that what you're doing will help you. Believing in what you are doing could be more important, or as important, as *what* you are doing. Additionally, you must put yourself in charge of your health. You already know that most medical doctors cannot help you. You must not relinquish control of your health to anyone; not even a MD. In order to believe in what you're doing, *you* have to be in control. Today, there are a number of different types of health practitioners. In addition to medical doctors, there are chiropractors, holistic practitioners, nutritionists, acupuncturists, massage therapists, and on and on. You may want to consult with more than one of these. You should view the MD, or any other health practitioner, as an assistant or counselor. You want their counsel and advice, but *you* make the final decision. I say this for a couple of reasons. First, medical doctors are not nutritionists. By the way, the life expectancy for a medical doctor is age 58. That statistic right there hardly qualifies him as an expert in longevity. Most MD's believe only in what they were taught in school and/or what they read that is hand fed to them by the American Medical Association. They are taught very little about nutrition. Most MD's think they have a corner on the health market, but contrary to their belief, they don't any longer. I read that in 1997 more people in the U.S. visited an alternative healthcare practitioner than those who visited their primary care physician. Secondly, MD's have really painted themselves in a corner. They have become very limited specialists dealing primarily with drugs and surgery. If they don't have a drug or a surgery for your ailment, then most of the time they can't help you. I believe drugs and surgery should be a *last resort*. Of course, if you break your arm, the MD is the right healthcare person to see. Additionally, if you have a urinary tract infection, a skin infection, or any disease treatable with an antibiotic, then again, your old MD is the person you want to see. I want to give the MD credit where credit is due.

Before I say too much more about the medical doctors, let me point out that my opinion is based largely on my own personal experiences and some experiences in my family. Here is an example of a family experience. When my mother was about 30 years old, she became very sick and was put in the hospital. Her doctor told my stepfather that he wanted to surgically remove one kidney that was inflamed. Fortunately, my stepfather did not approve and removed my mother from the hospital immediately. Of course, this upset the doctor considerably. My mother was taken to a different doctor and treated successfully without surgery. Many years later, my mother had a reoccurrence of the same problem. Medicine had advanced by that time and they discovered that my mother only had one kidney. Apparently she was born with only one. Now I don't have to tell you what the result would have been if my stepfather had not objected to that surgery. That immediately developed mistrust in my mind for doctors. I have had many more personal experiences with MD's over the years that were less than satisfactory. Now let's get back to ALS.

If you have ALS, you already know that most MD's can't help you as they have no effective drugs and no treatment. Therefore, if you have what I will call a *standard issue MD* then you have no choice but to divorce your MD and seek help from among the other alternative healthcare practitioners.

Positive mental attitude (PMA) and prayer have a place here also. PMA and prayer are the foundation for any improvement program.

To explain positive mental attitude or PMA, I must bring in my grandma. My entire family had PMA long before those three words were ever put together. My grandmother had a ranch north of Banning, California and when I was age three to ten; I spent my summers with my grandmother on that ranch. No one was more PMA than my grandma and she influenced me a lot. She would never let anyone, including me, get away with saying "I can't do this" or "I can't do that." She used to say, "There's no such word as can't." Let me tell you of one illustration. When I was about twelve and living in Hollywood, my grandma was visiting us for a time. One Saturday morning I was "hangin' a snoot." That's a family expression for being depressed. Grandma asked me, "What was the matter?" I explained, "All my friends are going up to Ferndell Park for the day and I can't go." (Ferndell Park was about three miles from my home.) She asked again, "Why can't you go?" I said, "My bicycle has a flat tire."

She said, "Well, you can walk can't you?"

I gave her a look as if she was out of her mind and said with great exclamation, "I can't walk all the way up there!"

Her reply was simple and clear, "Sure you can, you just put one foot in front of the other." Now that is a classic illustration of PMA. My grandma was "Mrs. PMA."

Here's how to make PMA work for you:

First, select a goal. Remember you can't have a dream come true, if you don't first have a dream. You may want both short-term goals and one long-term goal. You may want to restore your health as a long-term goal. You may want to increase the movement of your legs as a short-term goal.

Second, you must *believe* in what you're doing. (More on that in a moment.)

Third, you must *work* positively in the direction of your goal. Setting a goal and believing you can achieve it may work on its own. However, it is far more effective if you *work* toward your goal. Sometimes the accomplishment of the goal may not come directly from your effort. However, you have far less chance of meeting your goal without effort on your part. An important point here is to recognize that everything you do may not work. Therefore you must be flexible and change when this happens. If one thing doesn't work, then try another. Sooner or later you must find a way.

Napoleon Hill, who wrote *"Think and Grow Rich,"* said "Anything the mind can conceive and believe, it can achieve!" He was writing primarily about financial success and not health. However, I believe his slogan can be applied to health also. Remember, he said "Anything." Believing is the key word. If you don't believe you can do it, then you are most certainly correct; you can't. Now that you have selected a goal to restore your health, you simply have to work positively in that direction. I have personally used this formula for successful endeavors many times in my life. Let me give you just one example. One time when I was a recruiter, I set a goal to recruit 26 new people within six months. This was unheard of at the time. Most people in my position would recruit anywhere from five to ten a year. Well, I set my goal and worked at it. However, about five months down the road I only had about 19, way short of my goal of 26, with a month to go. I really kind of gave up, but I did keep working at it. Oddly enough, when the six months was up, I had recruited exactly 26 people. I can't really explain *how* it works; but it does.

Probably a far better example of PMA is the story of Thomas Edison. Even if you have heard this, it is worth repeating here and now.

The story goes that Thomas had done a thousand or more experiments trying to develop the light bulb. At that point in the story, he had not yet been successful, and a reporter from the local newspaper was interviewing him. The reporter asked Edison "Don't you feel like a failure having failed over a thousand times to develop your light bulb?" Mr. Edison replied "No, quite the contrary, I have proven successfully over a thousand ways that it won't work and I am that much closer to success." That may not be an exact quote, but you get the idea. Mr. Edison had a goal and he certainly maintained his PMA while seeking that goal. He must have *believed* all along that he would eventually succeed. This is also another example of Napoleon Hill and "Anything the mind can conceive and believe, it can achieve."

How do you develop PMA if you don't now have it? PMA begets success, or is it success begets PMA? It's the same question as "Which came first, the chicken or the egg?" Well, I don't know, but I do know that if you give me a chicken, I'll give you an egg, or give me an egg and I'll give you a chicken. PMA works the same way. Give me some PMA and I can be successful or give me some success and I will be more PMA. It's easy to have PMA if you're successful. Therefore, it is important that you recognize very early minor successes and build your PMA on that. In the beginning, you have to have PMA based on your faith and ability.

Now I don't want you to get the idea that I am "Harry Happy Face" all the time. I'm not. I get depressed just like anyone else in a similar situation. However, when I recognize depression, I remind myself to get back on the PMA. It is hard to have a so-called "terminal illness" and go around looking like "Sammy Smiley Face" all day. The important thing is to recognize when you are depressed and correct it by thinking PMA and put your "Sammy Smiley Face" back on.

Now let's talk about prayer.

Some people may not know how to pray. I'm not sure either, but I would like to share with you my thoughts on prayer. Let's assume you are a twelve-year old and you have no bicycle and you want one. I don't believe you should pray for God to provide you with a new bicycle. That may or may not work. My theory is to pray that He will show you the way to earn enough money to buy a new bicycle. That might work a whole lot better. When I pray, I always ask Him to show me the way to heal myself.

PMA and prayer have a lot of similarity in the way they work. They might even be the same thing with different names. When you pray, you are communicating with God. When you use PMA, you are communicating with your body intelligence. Again, they may be the same thing. Perhaps what I call the body's intelligence may be an extension of God: who knows? Another thing, you can't just pray once and forget about it. Neither can you select your goal and think PMA one day and forget about it. Both are ongoing, to be repeated day after day. You must pray everyday. You must think about your goal in a positive manner everyday.

Studies in hospitals have established that patients recover more often and quicker when they have people praying for them. Even the medical doctors are beginning to see the value of prayer in healing. If you don't believe in God or are skeptical, let me tell you a story about my dream experience that changed my entire attitude about God and prayer. I must first tell you something about me before the dream. When I was age five to twelve, we moved around frequently in the Los Angeles, California area and I attended whatever local church was available. I have attended more churches of different religions than most people. Many of them would tell me that if I did not believe in their particular religion, then I would go to Hell. Well, that didn't add up in my book so I became very 'un-religious.' From age thirteen, I was an Atheist. As I grew older, though, I became less certain and I would call myself an Agnostic. Then came the dream. Before I tell you about the dream, however, I must tell you the prelude.

My dad had died a few months or maybe a year before my dream. My dad had been an alcoholic for the last twenty years of his life and had borrowed money from me without repaying it many times. The worst thing, however, was when he borrowed my Colt 38 revolver. He never gave it back. I told him when he borrowed it that I had paid more for it than it was worth in any pawnshop, so please don't pawn it. Well, when he died, my brother took care of everything and asked me if there was any property of my dad's that I wanted. I asked him if he had my gun. My brother said yes he had a gun and I could have it. The thought that my dad still had my gun made me feel much better. However, that good feeling did not last long as I soon found out that it was not *my* gun. It was an older gun of far less value. Now this really crushed me. In fact, I was extremely hurt and mad at my dad. It really bothered me and I thought about it daily.

Then came the dream! It was what they call a psychic dream. I didn't know it at the time, but I read about psychic dreams a couple of years later and this dream had all the earmarks of a psychic dream.

In the dream, my dad appeared standing in front of me on the front lawn of a house that I had never seen before. He was standing near a large sycamore tree. My dad died of a stroke that affected one side of his body, and in the dream, he appeared with one arm in an emaciated condition. During the dream, the arm was restored to normal. My dad communicated with me by *thought transfer.* There were no spoken words. Now that is unique; I've never had a dream like that before or since. I normally have verbal conversations with people in a normal dream. After we communicated for a while on the front lawn, we went into the house, through a bedroom, and into a walk-in closet. Here we communicated more. He told me he was OK and even had a gun of his own. When the dream ended, I awoke and bolted upright in bed. It was 3:00 AM. My brain was *overwhelmed* with one single thought:

"My dad really never hurt anyone."

He did not tell me this in the dream. This was a feeling and thought that was in my mind when I woke up. Never in all my life have I ever awakened after a dream and sat up in bed. I just don't do that, and especially not at 3:00 AM. This thought that my dad never hurt anyone was so powerful I am unable to do justice to it in writing; it was simply overwhelming. Let me point out that the dream occurred over twenty years ago and to this day I can picture it and the thoughts quite vividly. One of the characteristics about a psychic dream is that you don't forget it as you do most all other dreams. That dream changed my attitude toward my dad so drastically that I find it difficult to this day to say anything bad about my dad. And that, friends, was the whole purpose of the dream, I think. I believe that my dad was sent back down to me, and appeared in that dream, because I was so troubled by him. He was sent to erase my ill feelings toward him. Let me tell you, that dream certainly did the trick. Now you can draw any conclusion you want, but my conclusion is that there is life after death and my dad revisiting me in a dream is proof of that. If you accept that premise, then it opens up a whole world of possibilities about God and the hereafter. Since the dream, I have read many more things that support my thinking about God. I am now convinced and therefore believe in prayer.

Now we have discussed prayer and PMA, but this whole idea needs to be amplified because it is so critical to your success in healing. You will recall that I said earlier, the body heals itself. If you question that, let's look back at what the father of all medical treatment said:

> Hippocrates wrote, "The natural force within each of us is that greatest healer of all."

Let's discuss *how* the body can heal itself. A crab can lose a pincher arm and simply re-grow one. Is that a miracle or what? A human can't do that but it can do something similar. You can break a bone and completely separate the two pieces, and yet when set properly they will grow back together. Isn't that a miracle too? You can cut yourself and many times when it heals there won't even be a trace. That too is a miracle in my book and hard to understand exactly how that works. Well, I think I have a clue for you. In order for the body to heal itself, there must be some form of intelligence at work . . . right? But where is the intelligence? Is your conscious mind directing these things? No it isn't. We know that. Is it your subconscious? Well, maybe. However, even if the subconscious is directing it, there is more to it than that. In the book *"Quantum Healing,"* the author Deepak Chopra MD, discusses this idea. Now here is a MD talking about the influence of the mind in healing. How encouraging!

In his book, Dr. Chopra asks the following question: How does one determine whether an object has intelligence or not? Here is the answer as I understand it.

This is determined by whether or not the object
has control over its own actions.

Now that is pretty interesting, at least to me. Let's explore that idea
some more. What happens when you cut yourself and some foreign
substance gets in the cut? Many white corpuscles rush to the cut to
attack the infection. I ask you now where is the intelligence that causes
this to occur? It could be that the brain is directing it. However, the little
white corpuscles have to know *what to do* when they get there, and
they have to *recognize* when they are there. Does that mean that they
are controlling their own actions? I think they must be. According to
the definition earlier on what is intelligence, the white corpuscles must
have it in order to do what they do.

Dr. Chopra's definition of intelligence explains a lot of things. That
means that not only does your body have a mind of its own, but also all
of your body parts have a mind of their own.

Another illustration involves red corpuscles. People who live at higher
altitudes have more red corpuscles. Red corpuscles carry oxygen. At
higher altitudes, there is less oxygen in the air, so the body creates
more red corpuscles in order to provide the body with more oxygen.
Let's think about that a minute. How does the bone marrow, where the
red corpuscles are produced, know to increase production when the
body is at a higher altitude? The conscious brain doesn't order it. The
subconscious brain might order it, but how does it know? This is clearly
an indication that intelligence is in all areas of our body.

I hope you're still with me and don't think I fell out of my tree! I do
hope you accept the idea that the red and white corpuscles must have
some form of intelligence on their own, in order to direct their individual
actions. If you don't, pause right now and think about it, or get the
book *"Quantum Healing"* and read it. Now the next step. What tells the
white corpuscles to go into action? I'm certain the subconscious brain
must have some control here. If you accept these ideas, and I hope you
do, then this explains how the body heals itself. Just like your breathing
is on automatic pilot, the body performs many functions without your

conscious brain directing it. We also know that all experiences of the conscious mind are transferred to the subconscious. Now we're getting to the heart of the matter. This is how, in my opinion, prayer and/or PMA work. All your positive (or negative) thoughts are transferred to your subconscious and influence all your body's actions or functions. It's just like a large company. The owner or president sets the tone. If he sets an example with a positive mental attitude, it will filter down throughout the organization.

To illustrate how the subconscious brain works, let me tell you a couple more stories. The first story is an experience I had when I was about fourteen. At that age, I slept like a rock. You could even fire a gun in the house and it wouldn't wake me. That is not an exaggeration, because my dad did that one night, and I never even knew about it 'till he told me the next day. No, he didn't shoot anyone; he was just target shooting into the back yard through an open window. Now, here is the rest of the story. My dad used to take me fishing on the pier in Malibu. Yes, fishing on the pier. You could even catch fish, big halibut, from the pier back in the 40's. The night before our first such fishing trip, my dad told me that we would go fishing the next day, *if* I would wake him at 4:00 AM. You see, we didn't have an alarm clock in those days. We weren't exactly poor, but not much better off than poor. Anyway, I can remember going to bed and thinking: "Boy, I just 'gotta' wake up at 4:00 AM." I thought that over and over and then fell asleep. This might be hard for you to believe, if you haven't done it, but I woke up at 3:55 AM. Is that another miracle of the mind, or what?

The second story about the subconscious has to do with memory. I read somewhere that if you try to remember something and you can't, then you do the following. Say to yourself, "I'll think of it later." By knowing what you want to remember, and telling your mind to relax now and that you will think of it later, you will. I have experienced this one many times since I first read about it. Many times the answer will occur within a few minutes. This is another example of PMA. Most people will say, "Darn it, I just can't remember that." That, of course, is what will happen; you won't remember. The positive approach is to say; "I will remember it."

Have you ever had a great idea suddenly occur to you out of the blue? If so, you have probably experienced what I just described, as this formula works well for problem solving too. You think about the problem clearly in your mind and then put it to rest. In time, the answer to the problem will surface.

"Eric, why are you making such a big thing about this?" Well, my thought is this. If you don't understand this, then you don't have a prayer. You must think positive. You must be happy. You cannot be depressed. This is why I said earlier "You must believe you can do it." You must reinforce yourself with positive thoughts and/or prayers everyday. Actually, you should find time at least once everyday, to concentrate on your goal through meditation and prayer. I believe that your conscious thoughts will be transferred and understood by the other intelligence in your body. It is a really big order to remain positive and not be depressed if you have a problem like ALS. Even though it is a big order, I know you can do it. I did it. If I can do it, I'm certain you can too!

Before we leave this subject, I would like to tell you one more story about my aunt Meda to emphasize the power of the mind. Meda was my mother's older sister by eight years. She was born in 1900. That made it easy for me to remember her exact age. My mother told me this story. She was there when it happened. When Meda was about 18 years old, she developed a very serious illness, either Diphtheria or something similar, and they weren't sure if she would live. Meda went into a coma. The doctor visited everyday and she had a 24-hour nurse. After a few days of no change in Meda's condition, my grandma told the doctor that if Meda wasn't better the next day, he was fired. This upset the doctor and he told my grandma that Meda might die. Well, the next morning Meda was not any better and grandma ordered the doctor and the nurse out of the house. My grandma then called in a Christian Science Practitioner (CSP). The CSP arrived that afternoon and sat up with Meda all night long. The next morning, Meda came out of her coma and in a few days was well. I don't mean to bring religion into this discussion; I only tell this story for its value regarding the power of the mind. As you may know, Christian Scientists believe in no treatment by any medical doctor. They believe in the power of the mind to heal.

Meda's experience caused her to become a devout Christian Scientist for the remainder of her life. Now here's the point of all this. Meda lived until 1998. Yep, you're right. She was 98 years old. Although that is a great accomplishment in itself, it isn't the main point. My aunt Meda, in all of the next 80 years, never saw a doctor, never took any medication, and never even took an aspirin. Is that remarkable or what? I don't know anyone else alive today who hasn't seen a doctor at some time in his or her life. I don't know what Meda would have done if she would have broken her arm, for example, but she never did. That too is remarkable. The power of the mind is awesome. We just don't know what all it can do. Let's not underestimate the power of the mind.

We have danced all around this body intelligence idea, so let's sharpen our focus.

You must *know*, and you need to *believe*, that the body has a mind of its own.

You must *know*, and you need to *believe*, that the body can heal itself.

You must *know*, and you need to *believe*, that *you* can influence your body's intelligence and healing process.

I offer you a couple of more stories that should be clinchers.

Body Has a Mind of Its Own

Throughout my lifetime, I have observed many fat people on many diets. Ninety-nine percent fail and here's why. Most people attempting to lose weight do so by reducing calories and basically starving their bodies to excess. I theorized years ago from my observations of these people that the body has a mind of its own.

The body says, "This person is starving me. Therefore, the next time I get a lot of food, I will turn it into fat and save it for future starvation periods. Further, I will be reluctant to part with any of that stored fat. I must save fat for the starvation periods."

It is obvious that this is what the body does. I have read recently that medical scientists have proven that this really takes place. It is further very obvious that the body does this on its own.

Conclusion: The body must have an intelligence of its own.

You Can Influence Your Body Health

I'll tell you something now that you and all medical doctors are aware of, yet the medical doctors don't really accept the idea. Here it is. You probably know what a placebo is, but just for clarification I will tell you. A placebo is a fake pill. It is a pill that looks like a prescription drug but has no drug content. From having done clinical trials on large numbers of people for years and years, medical science knows that the body heals itself and that your attitude can influence the healing. They know that when they give you a drug and tell you it may cure you, you may cure yourself in spite of the drug. In order to test drugs more effectively, they always do clinical drug trials in groups of two or more. One group gets the drug and one group gets the placebo. The group getting the placebo may have some improvement for the reasons discussed. Therefore, the group getting the real drug must do better than the placebo group.

Conclusion: When the body is tricked by you taking a placebo, it is influenced by your attitude and belief. This is genuine clinically proven evidence that your conscious mind can influence the health of your body. If you have any doubt now, I give up. No I don't, just kidding!

You must know and believe that the body has an intelligence of its own, the body can heal itself, and *you* can influence your own healing.

CHAPTER 4

PRE-ESTABLISHED BELIEFS

My health improvement program is very controversial and may involve a lot of new ideas to you. Before we go into my program, let's lay some groundwork for the acceptance of new ideas. If you are not open to new ideas, then you will never improve your ALS condition. The ideas discussed here are to help you or a caregiver to be open-minded to new ideas. Remember, your medical doctor has probably told you, as mine did, that there's no cure or treatment for ALS. Therefore, your only options are to go home and die *or* seek out *alternative treatments*. Let me mention that it is of equal importance that your caregiver be open to new ideas and alternative treatments.

In my mind, it is almost criminal that a medical doctor would tell you there is no treatment for ALS. There is much that can be done and you would expect any ALS doctor to know that there are some treatments available. Just as an example, clinical trials have proven that Vitamin E and Creatine can have a positive effect on the ALS condition. No, they alone won't cure ALS, but they can help.

There is much more that can be done, as you will see in later chapters. These two items are only examples.

Again, you need to be open-minded. I believe whole-heartedly in the following expression:

> "It's what you learn after you think you 'know it all'
> that really counts."

You don't want to be a know-it-all who is not open to new ideas. Someone once said, "Only the dead and the foolish never change their opinion." There is a dumb joke that goes like this: "Don't be so open-minded that your brain falls out." The joke has a point. However, that is the opposite extreme of being closed-minded and we don't want either extreme. The middle of the road is where I like to travel. I want to be open minded, but with a little bit of skepticism.

While we are talking about being open-minded or what one should do or not do, let me remind you that professionals built the Titanic. Who built the Ark?

When you have ALS, or some similar terminal illness, you are looking for help anywhere. That reminds me of one of my favorite expressions:

> "Do something, even if it's wrong!"

After all, what do you have to lose? It is time to do something even if you are wrong. It is time to question our pre-established beliefs and become more open-minded.

Over the last few years, I have learned some very interesting traits of human nature by observing a lot of different people and their reactions. One of them is our ability to totally disregard new hard evidence or new ideas when they conflict with our pre-established beliefs. This trait may be a defensive posture to avoid mistakes. Remember what P.T. Barnum said, "A sucker is born every minute." Nobody wants to be a sucker. But wait a minute, according to P.T. Barnum most of us are suckers. Well, that's true, at least some of the time, and here is the explanation. If we want to believe something, we can be fooled very easily. If we don't want to believe something, then we will reject it in spite of hard evidence to the contrary. A good example of the situation where we don't want to believe it involves a mother. The policeman is standing at the door telling the mother that her young son just robbed the liquor store. What's her reaction going to be? Nine times out of ten, it's going to be "My little Johnny wouldn't do a thing like that." It will take a volume of evidence to change her mind. An example of the opposite reaction is where you're told that you just won a million-dollar jackpot. It won't take much evidence to convince you because you want to believe that one.

In the recent past, I have written several articles that have been published in "*The ALS Digest*," an Internet newsletter which was published several times a week and e-mailed to 5100+ subscribers in 70+ countries. In case you may want to subscribe, here is the address:

This publication is apparently no longer available.

As a result of the many articles, I was able to make e-mail contact with many other PALS. I have learned a lot about ALS from them. I have also learned about one human frailty from some of the negative responses I have received.

The human frailty is **too much conviction in our pre-established beliefs.**

Before I go too far here, let me say that pre-established beliefs are very important to all of us. They are the backbone of our knowledge and attitude. However, I'm certain that none of us, including me, have pre-established beliefs that are 100% correct. Therefore, we need to question them occasionally.

Many of us have difficulty in valuing new information when it conflicts with our own pre-established beliefs.

There's a joke that goes like this:

"Don't confuse me with the facts; my mind is already made up."

My mother used to say "Many a truth is spoken in jest" and that joke is a beautiful example. I believe the O.J. Simpson verdict is another really good example of "Don't confuse me with the facts; my mind is already made up." Another example involves Santa Claus. You remember when you were a little kid and you believed in Santa Claus? Do you also remember the first time someone told you that there was *no* Santa

Claus? At first, you couldn't believe that there was no Santa Claus. Of equal importance you didn't want to believe that there was no Santa Claus. But, the truth is, there is no Santa Claus. I hope I haven't disillusioned anyone with this statement. What is the point of all this? Well, I want you to recognize that this human frailty exists. In seeking the truth, we must question our pre-established beliefs and be a little open-minded.

Let me tell you about two stories that really emphasize this human frailty.

Movies

Prior to 1930, we had only silent movies. There was no talking or any other sound. Someone, I'm not sure who, invented sound motion pictures or "talkies" as they were called then. The company with this new idea tried to sell it to every major studio in Hollywood and there were no buyers. Can you believe that? These people were so set on their pre-established ideas, that they could not conceive the value of this new idea. They finally sold the idea to a new up-coming film studio and you know the rest of the story.

Clocks & Watches

For years, the watch manufacturers in Switzerland had a corner on the market for quality watches and clocks. If it had a "Swiss Movement," it was quality stuff. One of the Swiss watch companies developed the digital clock and digital watch. They could not see the value of the digital clock/watch and felt that it would never amount to anything. Boy, were they wrong or what? Obviously, the digital clock/watch did not fit in with their pre-established beliefs, so they sold the idea to a Japanese company. You know the rest of the story. Do you know what the total sales of all digital clocks and watches have been since then? Well, I'm not going to tell you because I don't know either. You can rest assured that it is in the billions of dollars. This is just another example of our human frailty regarding the acceptance or denial of new ideas. Don't fall into that trap.

One of our pre-established beliefs is that the medical doctor is the last word. Let me point out that most medical doctors believe that too. Their attitude is that if a given procedure is not "proven," then it should not be used. However, their "proven" prescription drugs kill over 100,000 people a year here in the U.S. In a recent article in the newspaper, an HMO executive was quoted as saying that the figure is closer to 180,000.

History has shown us that the existing body of knowledge on a given subject can be wrong. Just because the mainstream thinkers say that it is so, that doesn't make it correct. It was only about 500 years ago that everyone in the world believed that the world was flat. That's one example of where the mainstream thinkers were wrong.

Here is a more recent one. Prior to the mid 1980's, the medical community was convinced that human brain cells were not reproduced. I guess that meant that when they all died, you did too. Now we know that's wrong. As brain cells wear out, they constantly reproduce at the rate of about 10,000 daily.

At one time about a hundred years ago, Congress wanted to close the U.S. Patent Office. Why on earth would they want to do that? Well, believe it or not, they thought all the possible new ideas or inventions had already been invented. "Eric, are you kidding?" No I'm not; that's the truth. That's about the epitome of denying or non-acceptance of new ideas.

Here's the point of all this. If you have ALS or some other medically untreatable disease, then you need to be open-minded to alternative treatments and alternative health practitioners. If you think that only medical doctors can help you, then you have a problem. Most medical doctors think that if a procedure is not AMA approved, then it must be non-effective or fraudulent and that *just ain't so*. If a procedure is not AMA approved, it may mean only that it hasn't been proven in a clinical trial. It does *not* mean that the procedure is not effective.

There is an old saying that goes something like this:

"None are so blind as those who refuse to look."

Many things I discuss in this book are controversial and they oppose mainstream medical thinking. However, that fact alone does not make them wrong. I'm here to tell you that I believe in everything I'm doing. I sincerely believe that I wouldn't be here if I hadn't done all of it. Everything I will tell you about has had some positive affect on my health.

All the above stories are meant to illustrate how pre-established beliefs can cloud your thinking. Please bear with me and let me tell you one more story that appeared recently in our local newspaper. This one is very sad, but it illustrates better than all the other stories, how dangerous pre-established beliefs can be:

> "New York – *FAULTY APPLIANCE LEADS TO SIX DEATHS*
>
> Six people were killed when an air conditioner absorbed carbon monoxide from a nearby furnace and pumped it throughout the house while they slept.
>
> Dr. Andrei Kranz, 46, discovered the bodies of his parents, his 2-year-old daughter, two house guests and a baby sitter Sunday morning. Kranz's wife and 17-year-old daughter were visiting relatives.
>
> Kranz later told police he had disconnected his home's carbon monoxide alarm because it buzzed repeatedly and he thought it was malfunctioning."

This is really a classic illustration of pre-established beliefs at work. Can you see it? The doctor was convinced that there could not be any carbon monoxide. That was a pre-established belief. He failed to accept the fact that the alarm was functioning properly. That was failure to accept evidence contrary to his pre-established belief.

I hope you see the reason and the need for all of us to question our pre-established beliefs now and then.

While we are on this subject, there is one more point to be emphasized. We are all a little spoiled by modern medicine. There is a pill for almost anything. It would be really neat if we had a pill for ALS. However, that does not now exist and in my humble opinion it may never exist. The treatment I put myself through to cure my ALS is not as simple and easy as taking a pill. For that reason, many people who are already skeptical will avoid the whole program. The program is not simple, but it works for me and I know several other PALS who have similar programs and it works for them too.

Well now, I have really talked a lot about pre-established beliefs and told you several stories. You might wonder why I have spent so much time on this subject. Frankly, I began wondering that myself. In a nutshell, I think that the number one reason is that too many people put too much faith in their medical doctor. Many people think that if a treatment was any good, their MD would know about it, and that just *ain't* right. No one doctor can know it all. Many medical doctors are guilty of having too much faith in their pre-established beliefs and their pre-established beliefs are limited to what they were taught in medical school or what they have learned from the drug companies.

Here is the second reason I spent so much time on this subject. I have learned that most people are not open to suggestions for their health improvement. It seems to be just the same as asking them to change their religion. Well, I guess most people are just not as open minded to health improvement ideas as I am.

Conclusion

I think it is imperative that you work with a healthcare professional who is open minded to alternative therapy. I am now working with a medical doctor who is specializing in alternative treatments such as chelation, hormone therapy, vitamins and other supplements, etc. Anyone living in my area of Southern California might want to consult with him. I have been seeing Dr. Rouzier for over six years now, and he has been a great help in my continuing improvement. Here is his name and information:

Neal Rouzier, M.D.
Preventive Medicine Clinics of the Desert
2825 Tahquitz Canyon Way, Suite B-200
Palm Springs, CA 92262
Phone (760) 320-4292

CHAPTER 5

TOXINS – POSSIBLE CAUSE OF ALS & OTHER CHRONIC ILLNESSES

Before we begin this subject, I feel the need for a little prelude. Some of you reading this, I'm sure, will question whether or not there can be so many toxins in our environment, which are harmful to us. After all, aren't the FDA and the government looking out for us? Yes they are, for the most part. However, they're not perfect. If you are like me, you may remember when you were seven, eight, or nine years old when you thought policemen were all 100% honest. Later, when you grew up, you were disheartened to learn that just *ain't* so. People are people no matter what their occupation and some are crooked, dishonest, and immoral. I don't mean to get real negative here, so let me be quick to point out that these are only a small percentage.

I'm sure you are also going to wonder why most medical doctors aren't aware of the problem with toxins. Well, medical doctors have a pre-established belief that evidence from clinical trials is the *only* evidence – period. They totally eliminate all anecdotal evidence of any kind. In many situations like neurological ailments, there are no clinical trials and there never will be. The *only* evidence we have is anecdotal; that is, stories about individual experiences. There are tons of individual experiences involving ALS and other health problems, which target toxins as the probable cause. Since this is the only medical evidence available, it is extremely shortsighted to not consider it at all. Anecdotal evidence is all we have to work with.

Thirty or forty years ago there were two health fanatics who each wrote several books on nutrition and health. I use the words 'health fanatics' because I don't know of any better words. I don't use it to belittle them; rather they are heroes in my opinion. Adele Davis died of cancer. This caused people to question whether her books on nutrition had any merit. Paul Bragge, on the other hand, died at the age of 95. He may have lived much longer if he wasn't killed in an accident. You might wonder why the difference in the outcome between these two. I believe that Bragge was more into avoiding toxins and detoxifying the body than was Adele Davis. I mention this only to establish the idea that nutrition alone may not prevent premature death and that avoiding toxins is equally or more important.

When I first began my program over seven years ago, I only had the general idea that toxins were at the heart of the problem. Since then, I have learned a great deal more. What I have learned has come from many different sources including many articles right from my local newspapers.

Here are some hard facts about toxins:

A Single Toxin Can Cause More Than One Illness

Tobacco, for example, can cause lung cancer as well as other illnesses like heart attacks and other circulatory problems. In the movie, "Erin Brockovich," (true story) several hundred people in one town developed tumors and many other illnesses from Chromium 6 which was in their drinking water. If you didn't see this movie, I would highly recommend that you do. The relationship of the many illnesses to Chromium 6 in the water was proven in court to the tune of a 333 million dollar settlement. I suggest that this is evidence that one toxin can cause more than one illness.

More Than One Toxin Can Cause the Same Illness

For example, tobacco is not the only toxin that causes lung cancer. There are many, many elements in our environment that are known to be carcinogenic. In plain language, that means they can cause cancer.

Now here's a puzzle for you. Even though most of us should realize that toxins cause cancer, when someone develops cancer, they still wonder where it came from. Why is there any surprise? In the last fifty years, the chemical industry alone has introduced some 75,000 new synthetic substances. The United States Government Center for Disease Control and Prevention reported the results of a recent study involving over 5,000 United States residents. They reported that the blood and urine levels of 27 different toxic chemicals were present in unexpectedly high levels. These chemicals are commonly found in soap, hair spray, nail polish, plastic products, etc. For example, a recent newspaper article stated that carcinogenic chemicals in permanent hair dyes could significantly increase the risk of bladder cancer when used over a long period of time.

Now let's discuss more about the relationship of toxins to illnesses. You may not realize it, but we are a sick country. A few decades ago, a country by country health survey was done and the United States was found to be eighteenth out of 119 countries surveyed. In a more recent survey of only 79 countries, guess where the U.S.A. was? You may have guessed it. We were in last place. Seventy-ninth! That means we are going downhill fast.

Half of all Americans today have one or more chronic illnesses. Yes, I said half or 50%. Additionally, four out of five of those, or 40% of the population, have *two or more* chronic illnesses. This information was developed by John Hopkins School of Public Health in Baltimore. Some of these 125 million people with chronic illnesses have only minor problems such as allergies, etc. However, 60 million others have more serious and multiple chronic conditions such as heart disease, Alzheimer's, cancer, arthritis and more. Question: What is a chronic illness? I believe it is anything that persists and for which the standard medical community has no cure or effective treatment.

Based on all this information about toxins, I believe it is reasonably safe to presume that toxins are the root cause of many, if not all, chronic illnesses. In fact, I believe we have an *epidemic* of toxic-related illnesses in this country.

Why then don't the medical doctors tell us about this? Let's explore that.

There was a recent television documentary that sheds some light on the medical doctors and their treatment of toxin-related illnesses. The name of the documentary was "Desert Storm Syndrome." They interviewed a large number of individuals who had been in Desert Storm and had various illnesses. They related how they were treated by the military medical doctors. It became quite evident, as the program progressed, that the medical doctors do not understand how toxins can cause illnesses. One reason is that they apparently have no laboratory tests that indicate the existence of, or prior exposure to, toxins. Further, the doctors seemed to be compelled to make a *diagnosis*, even when they really should be saying, "I don't know." In all the Desert Storm cases, the doctors would diagnose the problem as "post traumatic stress." Now, *ain't* that a crock?! After several years, the military and the doctors have finally done a 180-degree turnaround and admit that these illnesses are toxin-originated. I think that is criminal that it took them so many years to admit it. However, the point of all this is that doctors do not have any tests or any other means of properly diagnosing toxin-originated illnesses.

Now, let's get back to ALS and toxins. I believe it is safe to say that most toxins in our environment and in our food products are put there by large corporations. It may be that the leaders in these large corporations don't really believe that they are doing anything wrong. They may truly believe that the toxins put into the environment or into their food products are perfectly safe. This comes under the heading of "pre-established beliefs." Obviously, they don't want to believe that their products could be harmful. I'm sure they don't go out of their way to read anything that would indicate that their product is harmful. Of course there is a small percentage like we just discussed who just don't care. They are only interested in the "bottom line" which is of course **profit**. For example, how many years did the top corporate officers in the tobacco industry try to convince the public that tobacco was safe and non-habit forming? They didn't care if tobacco was safe or not, they just wanted to sell all they could. I think it's important for all of us to realize that this same attitude can and does exist in other industries.

Let's discuss *how* toxins may cause health problems. *Something* is causing an increase in certain illnesses. In the early 1900's, for example, most doctors never saw a patient with cancer. Cancer has been increasing at a rapid rate in the last one hundred years, and most people still don't know what causes it. There are many who believe, as I do, that the increasing toxins in our environment are the basic cause. Without question, there is an unusual parallel in the two. For an example of how the use of toxins is increasing, a recent newspaper article stated that the overall use of pesticide in California had jumped 40% from 1991 to 1998.

A pesticide is a poison or toxin used to kill pests: insects, rodents, etc. It is not logical that a pesticide that can kill insects is totally harmless to humans. It may not kill the human immediately, but that doesn't prove it is harmless. To the best of my knowledge, there are few, if any studies on the long-term effect of toxins on humans; that is the long-term effect of so-called safe amounts of toxins.

Not only do we not really know the long-term effect of any given toxin, neither do we know the accumulated effects of many toxins over a long time. In other words, the human body might be able to withstand the accumulated effects of a single toxin over a long period of time. But, can the human body stand up to the accumulated effects of many toxins over a long period? For example, most water companies allow a certain amount of arsenic in our drinking water. Then, dentists think that amalgams with mercury are safe. Also, the FDA thinks that a certain amount of pesticides, insecticides, and additives such as preservatives and taste enhancers (MSG) in our food are perfectly safe. But again, how many can we stand? I read somewhere that the FDA has approved over 28,000 different food additives that are not natural. Now, that is a lot.

Again, and I repeat, how much or how many can we tolerate? We have no idea about the accumulative effect of all toxins in our environment and no one, to my knowledge, is even looking at this problem.

I'll use myself as an example. In looking back over the ten years prior to my ALS, I realize now that I had exposed myself to many, many toxins:

*** The dogs and cats had flea collars.

*** I sprayed the yard frequently with toxins such as Roundup. We had two acres and I sprayed all the open areas with Roundup. It kills everything that grows.

*** I did a lot of spray painting on my dune buggies. My friend and I built two new dune buggies and rebuilt four others, so there was a lot of painting. Being "macho," I never wore a mask or filter. In this case, "macho" is another word for "stupid!"

*** We had automatic insecticide sprayers in the house. They were on a timer and sprayed every fifteen minutes.

*** Wasp spray was another thing I used. We had a number of wasp nests on the house and garage. I discovered this wasp spray that would spray out a stream of insecticide ten or more feet. I could literally shoot down these wasps out of the air. The stuff was so lethal it would kill them instantly and they would fall like a rock to the ground. As lethal as it obviously was, it never occurred to me to take any precautions. What can I say? Dumb huh?

*** Being into dune buggies, I was around a lot of gasoline vapors all the time.

*** I drove two hours everyday on the freeway, breathing everyone's exhaust fumes.

*** We did a lot of fishing, so we ate a lot of fish. Most of the fish were caught in the ocean off southern California. We now know that fish in this area are highly polluted with many toxins including mercury.

*** I drank a ton of alcohol, mostly beer from aluminum cans.

*** One day I stepped into the motorhome and smelled something strange. Sniffing like a bloodhound, I traced it to the refrigerator. I opened the door, stuck my head in, and inhaled deeply. Well, I was right, it was coming from the refrigerator, but the ammonia was so powerful it stopped my breathing. I literally could not breathe an ounce of air. The ammonia had severely burned my throat and lungs. I quickly walked out of the motorhome thinking that at least someone would find me when I passed out. Well, it wasn't as bad as I thought because

I began to breathe after about one minute. And now for my next "macho" trick! No, I don't think I'll do any more tricks like that one.

*** Last but not least is the prescription drug Flagyl. I think that was the final blow; like the straw that broke the camel's back, or maybe more like the redwood tree that broke the camel's back. More on Flagyl later.

Let's get back to toxins in our environment.

The same newspaper article that I mentioned previously, points out that "Metam Sodium" is a cancer-causing pesticide, and the use of that specific pesticide is up 400% in 1991 to 1998. That is really scary. Additionally, the article states that California's statewide use of pesticide amounts to 1.5 billion pounds in those years. Yes, that's right, 1.5 billion. Now that, friends, is a lot of poison.

There was another recent newspaper article on DDT and Chlordane. These highly toxic pesticides were banned many years ago. According to the article, scientists planted a garden in a field that had been treated with Chlordane 38 years before. Chlordane turned up in all twelve of the vegetables grown in that field. Please don't tell me that the continued and increasing use of pesticides is no threat to the human race.

My purpose here is to provide you with more evidence of how badly our environment is contaminated with toxins. For example, in one day in October 2000, the "Los Angeles Times" had three articles about three different toxins:

1. A blue food dye may have caused three deaths in Massachusetts. Three hospital patients received their liquid food containing the blue dye and their skin and blood turned blue hours before they died. Here is an example of toxic pollution in our food in a hospital. Is nothing sacred?

2. Another article is about Lockheed-Martin Corporation and contamination of the ground water in the area of their aircraft manufacturing plant in Burbank, California. The alleged contamination of soil and ground water covers a thirteen-mile area.

3. A separate article states that Chromium 6 levels are high in the tap water at 110 government facilities throughout Los Angeles County, California. Chromium 6 levels up to 8 parts per billion were reported. The recommended limit is .2 parts per billion.

In addition to the above, it was Chromium 6 that was at the heart of the pollution problem in Hinkley, California which was the basis for the movie "Erin Brockovich."

Let's talk about toxins and ALS, and when I say ALS I mean to include most any other similar nervous disorder like MS or Parkinson's. Eric, do you mean to imply that one toxin could cause more than one neurological ailment? Yes, that is exactly what I mean. The simple explanation is this. Whether you develop ALS or Parkinson's may be like the story of the chain and its weakest link. If you stretch the chain beyond its capability, you will break one link. Stretch it again and you'll break another but different link. I believe that we are all different and certain areas of the nervous system may be stronger or weaker in one person than in another.

ALS is difficult to diagnose. For one reason, there is no single test for ALS. Many PALS have been misdiagnosed in their early stages of development. When all you have are one or two symptoms, ALS can be confused with many other neurological illnesses. Frequently Lyme disease is misdiagnosed as ALS. It is caused by the bite of a tick. There really shouldn't be any confusion between Lyme and ALS. Lyme can have as many as 40 symptoms almost all of which are different from ALS symptoms. The only common symptom I see is muscle weakness and paralysis.

There's a very interesting article in the June 16, 2003, issue of "People Magazine." It's a story about a man who was mistakenly misdiagnosed for ALS and later found out he had Lyme disease.

In my opinion there's no reason for this to happen because many symptoms of Lyme are very different from ALS. However, misdiagnosis is a major problem. This man in the article was 34 years old and suffered from high blood pressure, double vision, facial palsy, fatigue, and joint pain. Additionally, his body weight went from 307 to 202. Now I might be wrong, but I think the only two real ALS symptoms of his were fatigue and loss of weight. Still, however, he was misdiagnosed. The article said his doctor really didn't know what to do and kept referring him to other doctors.

Now here is a very interesting point. A friend, not a doctor, questioned the symptoms and suggested he see a Lyme specialist, a Dr. Greg Bach in Philadelphia. Dr. Bach found a rash beneath the patient's hair that obviously all the other doctors had overlooked.

The point of all this is that Lyme disease is misdiagnosed often and Lyme is treatable and ALS is not. I believe that any one of you out there who has been diagnosed with ALS should review the symptoms and consider consulting with a Lyme specialist; not just any doctor, but a Lyme specialist.

Caution – Lyme Treatment

According to information I have received, you should not take minocycline. The British Journal of Medicine states that minocycline can cause liver failure, Hepatitis, and Lupus. This could be deadly for an ALS patient. Many doctors prescribe this drug for treatment of Lyme disease. That's wrong. Lyme disease was originally classified as a virus and it still is a virus. It has been reclassified as bacteria and, again, that's wrong.

Colloidal silver is a suggested treatment and it should completely eliminate the Lyme virus with no bad side effects.

For more information on Lyme, go to the Internet.

I know I said earlier that it didn't matter which toxin caused your ALS condition because the treatment is still the same. However, I feel compelled to discuss that more thoroughly in an effort to convince you that my theory is correct. There are many people who believe toxins cause ALS and most of us have developed our theory independently of the others. I say this because I don't want you to think that I am the Lone Ranger here. For example, read the book "The Brain Wellness Plan" by Dr. Jay Lombard and Carl Germano. Dr. Lombard is a Board Certified Neurologist and according to his book he believes in the toxin theory as I do. Also read the book "Toxic Metal Syndrome, How Metal Poisonings Can Affect Your Brain" by Dr. H. Richard Casdorph and Dr. Morton Walker.

First of all, there are other neurological conditions that are known to be caused by toxins. There is a condition with no specific name called simply "Iron Overload Syndrome." This condition is clearly caused by a heavy metal. By the way, you should be tested for this and it requires a special test. There are many other neurological diseases similar in some ways to ALS. There is Multiple Sclerosis, Parkinson's disease, Alzheimer's, etc. I believe most of these and possibly all of them are caused by toxins.

If you are teetering on the edge of belief or disbelief on toxins, here is a story that could be a clincher. There was an article in the "*Philadelphia Inquirer*" about a chemical fire that occurred twenty years ago. It seems it had caused many health problems. One story goes like this: Two men, who walked side by side collecting chemical samples during the fire, died of ALS within fourteen months of each other.

There is still another story I need to tell you about. I've read this story two or three times from different sources. There was a nurse who apparently fell while carrying a thermometer. The thermometer broke and penetrated her hand injecting some of the mercury into her system. Within a short time, she developed ALS.

No single story like these proves anything. However, I have heard many similar stories involving mercury, amalgam fillings, and pesticides. Even though they don't in themselves prove anything, I don't believe they can be ignored either. There are way too many of them. It seems to me that the coincidence of toxins and ALS is too great to be a mere matter of chance. If you believe in coincidence, then you do not want to apply for a job as a detective.

There are many physical ailments, in addition to neurological diseases, that can be traced to toxins and particularly heavy metals. Again, read the book "*Toxic Metal Syndrome*" previously mentioned. One example in that book is mercury. These two medical doctors believe that Alzheimer's is caused by mercury and other heavy metals. They claim to have cured thousands of Alzheimer's patients with chelation therapy and removal of amalgam dental fillings. It is well documented that mercury causes many other health problems. It is my belief that mercury is involved in ALS to a large degree.

There is a *cause* of ALS. That fact is indisputable. ALS is not just old age. The reason that we haven't discovered the cause could be that we're overlooking something previously considered. **Mercury** could very well be that 'something' that we are overlooking. Here is the reason why. When mercury gets into your system, it finds its way into and attaches to your muscles and organs. A normal blood test may not indicate any mercury. However, if you get a hair analysis, it will indicate how much mercury you have in your system. You can get a hair analysis done by Great Smokies Diagnostic Lab, 63 Zillicoa Street, Asheville, NC 28801 (phone 828 253-0621). Normally, you have to get a hair analysis kit from a health practitioner. The hair analysis is an elaborate report. It will provide you with a report on all the heavy metals and minerals in your system. This will provide you with a guide to your supplement program. A periodic hair analysis will tell you of your progress.

The hair analysis is a good idea but if you're concerned more with mercury than anything else, then you should have two or three treatments of chelation therapy with DMPS, followed by a test of your urine. The chelation therapy must be done by a doctor and, if you are wondering what DMPS is, he will know. (There is more information about chelation with DMPS in Chapter 8.) I can almost guarantee that the urine analysis will contain mercury; that is assuming you have ALS and several amalgam dental fillings.

An amalgam is a dental filling made with 50% mercury, 35% silver and 15% other metals.

> **Note:** Since there is more mercury than silver, why do they call them silver fillings? Gee! You don't suppose they are trying to hide something do you?

Since mercury is our main concern of all the toxins, here are some more facts about mercury, amalgams, and our health:

1. Mercury is highly toxic. It is one of the most toxic metals known to man; second only to uranium.
2. Mercury poisoning can cause numerous health problems.
3. Mercury poisoning most commonly affects the nervous system.
4. Mercury is the number one **neuro**toxin.

5. Mercury has the ability to penetrate the blood/brain barrier and damage the motor neurons.

6. It is illegal for paint to contain mercury or lead. Why is it illegal to put mercury in paint, but legal to put mercury in your mouth in the form of a dental filling? Answer: **It should not be legal.**

7. Prior to placing the dental amalgam filling in your tooth, the material is considered hazardous material. When amalgam dental fillings containing mercury are removed from your teeth, they must, by law, be treated as hazardous waste material.

8. Tests have proven that the average mercury amalgam filling releases mercury vapor at the rate of about 10 mcg of vapor everyday and the body absorbs at least 10% of that.

Note: The American Dental Association would have us believe that this hazardous material is only hazardous before and after, but when it's in your mouth, it is perfectly safe. If you believe that, I would like to sell you some beach front property in Arizona.

Here is a brief history of the dental amalgam:

1830 – Dentists first started using amalgam dental fillings sometime between 1830 and the 1850's. Different sources give different dates.

1850 – The National Association of Dental Surgeons was opposed to the use of mercury amalgams. However the dentists continued to use them.

1860 – ALS was first diagnosed in the 1860's

Note: The use of mercury amalgams came first. Then, several years later, the first case of ALS was diagnosed.

1899 – The dentists formed a new dental association named the American Dental Association (ADA) and the old National Association of Dental Surgeons was dissolved. The newly created ADA approved of the mercury amalgams.

1920 – A prominent German chemist, Alfred Stock, proves that amalgam fillings leached out mercury and that the mercury caused many health problems.

1979 – Scientists at the University of Iowa proved that a measurable amount of mercury vapor is constantly being released from mercury amalgams.

1980 – Hal Huggins published his book about the dangers of amalgams fillings and root canals.

1990 & 2000 – Currently mercury amalgams are illegal in several foreign countries and laws have been passed in several states of the U.S. limiting their use or requiring a warning to consumers. There are many, many books written by medical doctors, dentists and other health professionals for the sole purpose of warning the public about the dangers of mercury. There are many doctors and dentists together with attorneys working to eliminate the use of amalgams.

I have access to a book that's about 8 ½ x 11 inches and over one inch thick titled "*Toxicological Profile for Mercury.*" It is a U.S. Government report published in 1998 by the U.S. Department of Health & Human Services, Public Health Service, Agency for Toxic Substances & Disease Registry. This report tells you everything you'd ever want to know about mercury. Most significantly, it states clearly that the major sources of mercury poisoning in humans are fish and dental amalgam fillings. Here is an actual quote from the report:

"A primary source of mercury exposure for many populations is through the consumption of methylmercury-contaminated fish and shellfish. Another common source of human exposure to mercury is dental fillings that contain metallic mercury as part of the amalgam. That such exposure can contribute to the existing body burden of mercury has been well documented in the scientific literature, but whether such exposure by itself presents a significant health risk is still a matter of some scientific discussion."

What could be clearer than that? A United States government report that says amalgams are unhealthy. In spite of that, there are numerous people, including doctors and dentists, who insist that amalgams are safe.

That last sentence in the quoted paragraph above may leave you scratching your head. All that means is that in spite of all indication that amalgams are unhealthy, it has not been accepted by the medical and dental community. Well, if you have a health problem such as ALS that could be related to mercury, I don't believe you can afford to wait for a final decision. In my opinion, if you have ALS and dental amalgams, you're "gonna die." If you have the amalgams removed, then you have a fighting chance. If I'm wrong, you have lost a few hundred dollars replacing your fillings. However, if I'm right, it may save your life. It's your choice and your funeral.

I don't expect you to just take my word for the fact that amalgam dental fillings with mercury are a health hazard. Therefore, I offer the following recent events.

According to what I read, there are three countries in Europe that banned the use of mercury in dental fillings.

The state of Maine, USA, recently passed a law requiring dentists to notify their patients that mercury amalgams pose certain health problems.

An organization called the National Black Caucus of State Legislators passed a resolution dealing with the health affects of mercury dental fillings. The resolution calls for changes in the state laws on:

1. Health warnings to all consumers.
2. Heavy emphasis on health affects on children.
3. Changes in private insurance funded by the state for the poor and moderate-income consumers so that they might choose other types of fillings.

A new California law effective in 2002 disbands the Dental Board of California. In other words, they fired the whole board including the leader. I read an article that explained why. According to the article, the board was not consumer oriented. Well, folks, that smells to me like mercury is involved. I don't know that, but I'd bet you a dollar it is.

I think the above events would adequately support the idea that there must be some solid evidence that mercury dental fillings are hazardous to your health; and that is putting it mildly.

In my personal survey of over 100 PALS, all but six had dental amalgam fillings. Here are the exceptions:

1. Retired 70-year-old male with all gold fillings – former occupation dentist.
2. 45-year-old female dental technician.
3. 55-year-old male dentist.
4. 60-year-old male – former greens keeper of a golf course for over 20 years. He did all the insecticide spraying which contained mercury.
5. 50-year-old male with no amalgams and yet tested positive for mercury and no obvious occupational exposure. He told me, however, that he "ate a lot of fish" and he said further "when I say a lot of fish, I mean *a lot* of fish!"
6. 58-year-old male who owned his own business selling agricultural supplies. It is my best guess that he was exposed to the vapor from insecticides containing mercury.

Note that none of the six people had amalgam dental fillings but all had ALS. Plus they all had an exposure to mercury from another source. All six of these people have lived longer than the average PALS. It may be because the source of their mercury exposure has been eliminated. That is unlike the people who still have mercury amalgams in their mouths.

Let me restate this to make it clear. Every PALS that I have surveyed had or has amalgam fillings or they are one of the six listed PALS who had mercury exposure from another source. In other words, 100% of all surveyed had exposure to mercury from one source or another.

I first got started on this amalgam theory while e-mail communicating with another PALS who had done a lot of research on amalgams. I wrote to him and indicated I only had two amalgam fillings. He was in his 40's and had 20 amalgams. He told me I was much older than he was. This startled me. How did he know how old I was? We had never met. I was 68 years old at the time. Now, here he was in his 40's with ALS and 20 amalgams while I, on the other hand, was in my 60's with only two amalgams. The obvious theory is, the more amalgams the sooner you get ALS. I decided to check this out. The first person I thought about was another PALS named Joe, whom I had met on the Internet. I knew Joe was over 60 and had ALS for 10 years with no special health program. I thought, "He must have fewer amalgams than I have." I contacted him and he told me he had one amalgam. Is that strange or what? I frequently ask other PALS about the number of their amalgams and their age. Everyone I have asked has confirmed my theory. That is, the age of onset is relative to the number of amalgam fillings. Additionally, the greater the number of amalgam fillings one has, the faster the progression of ALS symptoms.

I know the relationship of health and amalgam dental fillings is highly controversial. If you question any of this, I invite you to take your own survey among PALS. Just start asking other PALS about amalgams and I'm certain you will find the same results I did.

Additionally, DAMS, Inc. offers about 45 or more books and videotapes on amalgams, root canals and health issues. That's pretty impressive, isn't it? Most of these books are written by dentists and medical doctors. DAMS, Inc. full name and address is as follows:

DAMS, Inc,
Dental Amalgam Mercury Syndrome
P.O. Box 7249
Minneapolis, MN 55407-0249 USA
Phone 1-800-311-6265

DAMS, Inc. also has available a report with a wealth of information. Call them at the phone number shown above and request their "information kit." The information kit will include 20 pages of vital information about amalgams, root canals, gum infections, and their relationship to health problems. Their report also includes information about chelation treatments as well as very **specific instructions on how to safely remove mercury fillings.** They will also provide a list of healthcare practitioners in your area, most of which are dentists.

If you are seeking more information about anything related to amalgams, then there are two books that you should read:

"It's All in Your Head" by Dr. Hal A. Huggins

"Reversing Chronic Disease - Getting Well Again" by Tom Warren

These books will convince you as they have me that if I needed a root canal tomorrow I would not have that procedure done. I would have the tooth pulled and replaced. If you are a PALS and already have some teeth with root canals, then in my opinion, they should be removed. Dr. Huggins will explain why the Periodontal Ligament must be removed along with the root canal tooth.

If you would rather go to the Internet rather than read books, then you might view these websites:

> http://www.toxicteeth.org
> http://neuraltherapy.com/articles.asp
> http://www.neautaltherapy.com/hfiles/Mercury
> %20Detoxification.htm http://www.xs4all.nl/~stgvisie/
> AMALGAM/EN/SCIENCE/bernie_science.html
> http://dmoz.org/Health/Alternative/Non-Toxic_Living/
> Mercury_and_Amalgams/

If you're looking for holistic or biological healthcare practitioners for cavitational surgery, metal free dentists, you may want to view the following website:

> http://www.DentalHelp.org

Now you're going to ask a number of questions. First, "Why doesn't everyone with amalgam fillings get ALS?" My answer is a question: "Why doesn't everyone who smokes tobacco get lung cancer?" The truth is, I don't know the answer to either question. However, I believe that if you live long enough with a mouthful of amalgam fillings, you will eventually get ALS or some other neurological disorder. I have read that doctors estimate that if you live to be 85 you'll have a 50% chance of having Alzheimer's by then. That in my mind has to prove that toxins in our environment are causing this.

Second, I've heard of people having all their amalgams removed, but they did not get well. Why not? The answer is simple and obvious. *The simple removal of amalgams may not in itself cure you.* You've had the amalgams in your mouth for perhaps 20 or 30 years and the mercury is now in your system. You can't undo that overnight. Mercury attaches to muscle tissue and vital organs. The mercury must be removed from your system before you can get well. Also, now that you have ALS, your body is in a weakened condition and *other toxins* may be harmful to you.

The body has a lot of safeguards to protect your health. One of them is called the "Blood/Brain Barrier." There is a protective shield around your motor neuron brain cells to protect them from the normal amount of toxins in your system. However, nothing is perfect. This barrier can be worn out by excessive toxins, making your motor neuron brain cells susceptible to damage by *any* and *all toxins*. Therefore, even if you remove your amalgams and remove all the mercury from your system, you still might not get well unless you establish a program of *avoiding all toxins.*

This reminds me of a letter to Ann Landers that was presented in her column recently. A man wrote to her stating that he had developed Multiple Chemical Sensitivity. He stated that he had worked in a perfume factory for over ten years and he was convinced that caused his ailment. He would react to laundry detergent, perfume, anti-perspirants, hair spray, and more; even car exhaust fumes. He developed stroke-like symptoms, numbness, slurred speech, dizziness and nausea. This is an obvious example of how damage to your system caused by one toxin can make you more susceptible to damage by many more toxins.

Avoiding all toxins is a huge order. Actually, it can't be done a 100%. However, you must avoid all toxins possible and certainly the major ones. There will be more on this later.

We tend to underestimate the serious threat that these toxins create, and before we leave the subject of toxins, I have three stories for you. They are included to indicate how serious these toxins are and how we underestimate them:

*** The older brother of a long-time friend of mine retired from the Palm Springs Police Department. He was living in Northern California and his home had a beautiful outside sundeck. He decided to refinish the deck and spent all one day painting it on his hands and knees. He died five days later. I don't understand exactly what happened, but apparently the breathing of the vapors from whatever material he was painting with, damaged his lungs severely, so he was not getting adequate oxygen.

*** The second story is about my neighbor to the rear of my home in Mission Viejo, California. One windy day my neighbor bought some ant poison in the form of a yellow powder. He sprinkled it all around the base of his home. Apparently he breathed a great deal of the powder due to the wind that day. At any rate, it destroyed his brain.

*** A third story I read in a magazine. It seems that the wife came home and found her husband in his chair in the living room. He was alive but in a coma. The car was in the garage and no indication of what happened to him. Finally, they discovered the car ignition was turned on and the car was out of gas. The only probable explanation was that he came home, drove in the garage, and shut the door leaving the engine running. He was then overcome by the exhaust fumes of the car, but was able to stagger inside and fall in his chair.

These three stories should emphasize the seriousness of these toxins that we play with everyday.

There's one more thing I would like to tell you about to establish a clear relationship between toxins and ALS.

I worked many years for a large insurance company. The company had a very clever procedure or formula for problem solving. Whenever a serious problem occurred, we were asked to do a PCST. That stands for *problem, cause, solution,* and *timing.* Following this formula will cause you to analyze each of the four factors very carefully. You must have a clear understanding of the problem before you can go any further. Then, you must know the precise cause before you even think about any solution. Too often we think of a solution for a problem without really knowing the true cause. Too often that leads to an incorrect solution.

Let's apply this to ALS. You might think that the problem is that you have ALS. That's wrong. The problem is your muscles won't move and they are atrophying. Now that we have the problem clearly understood, let's go on to the cause. You might think that we don't know the cause. Wrong again. We do know a little bit. We know that the cause of ALS is that the motor neurons are dying. When they die, then no messages are sent to the muscles. Sometimes we have to look for the cause of *a cause* to solve the problem. That's the situation with ALS. The next logical question is "What is causing the motor neurons to die?" I'm not a medical scientist, so that might be good because I can deal only with generalities. The generality here is that something is killing the motor neurons, but what? It would almost have to be something toxic to the motor neurons. This may sound overly simplistic, but I think it's just that simple. What else would kill them if not a toxin? The motor neurons have a protection called the blood/brain barrier that the creator of the human body put there to protect them from *run-of-the-mill* toxins. Therefore, the toxin or toxins that are getting through the barrier must be very potent or they have been in the system a long, long time. Now, what kind of a toxin would attack motor neurons? It would be a neuro-toxin like mercury or monosodium glutamate. We're now ready for the solution. I will give you that in a later chapter, but obviously it is eliminating any and all toxins that might damage motor neurons.

The last item is timing. That's the easiest one of all. Start at once!

I hope that helps convince you of the relationship between toxins and ALS and other chronic illnesses.

Update – May 2004

Here are my latest thoughts about the cause of ALS. First, let me point out that the Muscular Dystrophy Association and the Jerry Lewis annual telethon have collected millions of dollars for research on the many neurodegenerative diseases like MD, MS, ALS, etc. Last year 2003 they were pledged to receive over 60 million dollars. Now folks, they have been doing this for over 50 years. Think about that a minute. Millions upon millions have been spent with no concrete results. I'm sorry to say this, but I really wonder if they are misdirected or perhaps they just do not want to find the answer. A cure for ALS would sure put a lot of people out of work who are now receiving those millions of dollars. Let's play Sherlock Holmes and look at this problem in the simplest way.

Here is the first question you might ask: Is the cause of ALS environmental or an infectious disease? The fact is the average age at onset of ALS is 54 which would seem to indicate environmental.

The second question: Since ALS is a **neuro**degenerative illness, what element could cause it? The first element on the list is mercury. Mercury is the number one neurotoxin.

Next question: Does mercury exist in our environment? The answer is a giant yes! Mercury is spewed into the air from many industrial plants throughout our country. Mercury is in most of the fish that we eat. Mercury has been used as a dental filling for 150 years. Mercury has been used as a preservative in many shots that are given to adults and children and that includes flu shots.

The above would make mercury my number one choice as a highly probable cause of ALS.

If a drug were to be created today that would cure ALS, that news would make headlines. But, if I told you that a drug has already been created for that purpose, not many would listen. In my opinion, that drug has already been created. It is called DMPS. It is a drug approved by the FDA for eliminating mercury from your body.

As Sherlock Holmes would say, "Elementary, my dear Watson, elementary."

CHAPTER 6

THE BEGINNING OF ALS–
1990 thru 1996

Now, let's go back before my diagnosis in 1996. In fact, we'll go all the way back to the real beginning of my story on ALS starting in 1990.

Like most PALS, I was very active outside of work. I water-skied, hunted, fished and rode a dirt bike in the California deserts. I also jogged three miles every morning before work Monday through Friday. Glenna and I both played racquetball twice a week. I shot a 500-pound elk in Colorado and packed out half of it on my back in 1988. Of course, it took me two trips to carry out one-half of it. My two buddies carried out the other half. I was 59 years old then.

I also had an off-road race dune buggy. I didn't race it, but we used it for pleasure trips. Several friends of mine had them too. Four of the couples, including Glenna and I, planned a week long dune buggy trip in Baja California, Mexico in April of 1990. A few days before we were to leave, it looked like Glenna and I would not be able to make the trip. I don't remember why now but I'm sure it was work related. The other three couples left on the trip Thursday night. Late Friday, it looked like we could get away after all, but were we too late? We thought about it and then figured a way to catch up with the other couples. The plan was to tow the buggies to Bahia de Los Angeles (Bay of L.A.), in Mexico, and take the buggies from there. We knew that on the second night out of the Bay of L.A., which was Sunday night, our friends would be in San Ignacio. Because they would be traveling in sand washes and rugged dirt roads, we figured we could drive the dune buggy on the highway from Bay of L.A. to San Ignacio and catch up with them. We knew this was a long shot. How would we find them in San Ignacio once we got there? We didn't know the answer to that one, but here's what happened. We were driving down the highway coming into San Ignacio and we had our CB radio on. Suddenly, we heard familiar voices speaking in English. Lo and behold, it was our friends headed out of town looking for a junkyard to find a replacement part for one of the buggies. I kept silent on the radio until they saw me. You can't believe their surprise.

Is this another example of PMA or what?

We had a great time on that trip! We continued on a big loop through all the back country of Baja and returned to the Bay of L.A. the following Saturday. Sunday we towed our buggies home. After we were home a few days, I developed chronic diarrhea. Well, that isn't unusual for having been to Mexico. However, my case was unusual. After testing many stool samples, it was finally determined that I had amebic dysentery. The actual name of the bug was Endamoeba Histolytica and it is as bad as the name sounds. If not treated properly, it is life threatening. The cure is terrible. They use a drug called Flagyl. Flagyl is a poison and highly toxic. It makes you so sick you can't believe that it is a cure. The only cure prior to Flagyl was arsenic. You had to take this poison to kill the bug and hopefully the bug would die before you did! You have probably guessed by now that medical doctors are not among my most favorite people. Well, here is one experience that will tell you why. I went to see four different medical doctors over a three-year period. Each doctor would recommend Flagyl, but the first three times it did not kill the bug. Then, now get this, I went to the Orange County Health Department (OCHD) and there I visited a doctor who really knew about Endamoeba Histolytica.

Here's what he told me:

> Take 750 mg Flagyl three times a day for ten days.
> Take 650 mg Odoxin three times a day for twenty days.

These must be taken in sequence and *never* at the same time. None of the other doctors had given me this precise formula. They had me take Flagyl alone or Flagyl and Odoxin at the same time. I went back to my last doctor with the information I had received from the *free service* at OCHD. When I told my doctor what OCHD said, his reply was "It won't make any difference." Can you believe his arrogance? I said emphatically "I want to do it anyway. We must do something different from what we have done." I followed the Orange County formula and I got rid of the bug. How about that! The *amateur* wins again.

I started the above story with the buggy trip so you could see how close I came to avoiding all this. If I hadn't gone on the buggy trip, I might not have had dysentery, I wouldn't have taken Flagyl, and I might not have developed ALS. Oh well, that's life!

They say there is never anything so bad that there isn't some good in it. Perhaps you will see some humor in this story about my visit to OCHD. A friend had referred me to OCHD because another friend of his had a similar problem to mine and when his medical doctor couldn't help him, he found relief at OCHD. I called them for an appointment. After a long discussion, the lady on the phone said somewhat reluctantly, "Well, come on in . . . . I guess we will treat you." I didn't understand this at the time, but you'll understand in a minute. I arrived at OCHD and was directed to the waiting room. My first impression was the seriousness of everyone in there. This was certainly "Somber City!" After the usual wait, a man in a white coat called me into his office and began asking me a lot of questions such as "With whom do you have sex?" "Do you have sex with women?" "Do you have sex with men?" "Do you have sex with both?" Now there is an interesting question! I didn't understand all this, but I went along with it. Then he told me to wait in the waiting room again. Soon, I was ushered into another office to see "The Doctor." He began reviewing all the sex questions. At this point, my curiosity was overwhelming and I asked him "Why all of the *sex* questions?"

He replied "You are in the VD Clinic!!!"

Yes, VD as in Venereal Disease. I still didn't get it and I asked "Am I in the wrong place?" He laughed and said no. I asked why am I being treated in the VD clinic? He said I had a sexually transmittable disease.

I still didn't get it and I asked "How do you figure that?" He said "Well you know how the guys do *it*." Finally, the dawn came! It had never occurred to me that having amebic dysentery could be a sexually transmittable disease. Good thing they look at it that way, otherwise I might still have that Endamoeba Hystolitica bug.

"Eric, what does all this have to do with ALS?" Well, it was shortly after this that I began to develop ALS symptoms. As you know, I believe ALS is caused by toxins. Flagyl is toxic. I believe taking Flagyl four different times was much more than anyone could normally handle without some serious adverse affects. Also, many PALS have physical traumas related to the onset of ALS. I'm certain that this entire experience, including having diarrhea for three years, was traumatic to my system.

Here's another one on medical doctors. At this point in time, I still had diarrhea even though the Histolytica bug was gone. I asked my new doctor, I'm now on number five, what to do about my diarrhea. You won't believe what he said. He said "Take Imodium anti-diarrheal caplets." Well, I didn't take his advice because that sounded like a temporary solution to a long-term problem and incorrect. Instead, I found a nutritionist and colon hydrotherapist. She recommended an herbal pill. She suspected I still had some other bugs in there. I took the herbal pills as directed and my diarrhea stopped. What a relief!

The name of the herbal remedy is "Para-Cleanse" by Nature's Sunshine Products, Inc. 1(800) 223-8225. This product is available at most health food stores and instructions are on the package.

This is a good place for a joke about medical doctors:

"What is the difference between God and a medical doctor?"
Answer: "God does not think he is a doctor."

Don't get me wrong . . . there are some good medical doctors. The problem is there are not enough. There are many, many medical doctors who are getting into alternative care treatment and I admire those who are broadminded enough to do that. Perhaps in the future more of them will follow suit.

Recognize in the above story that the medical doctors did not cure my diarrhea but the alternative care person did cure it.

My first ALS diagnosis was by a medical doctor in late 1993. After all the tests were done and the diagnosis was in, I remember his nurse calling me to arrange another appointment. I recall asking her why the appointment? Could the doctor do anything to help me? She said no (of course). At that point I said, "Well then, there won't be any need to make another appointment."

I selected a doctor (Osteopath) who specialized in "alternative treatments" such as chelation therapy and hyperbaric oxygen treatment. I enjoyed working with him. He's the one who later on told me I had to make my body as pure and *pristine* as possible by avoiding toxins. *Pristine* was a motivating word. That's what got me started on my program later on in 1996. My program is discussed in Chapters 7, 8, and 9. When I first started with him around 1993, he didn't tell me to avoid any and all toxins. He did tell me to eliminate coffee and alcohol at that time, but I just couldn't do it. He did start me on a very comprehensive vitamin regimen. I was taking about ten or more vitamin tablets or capsules with each of three meals daily. The regimen included the following:

Vitamin E – 3600	B Complex – 50
Vitamin B1 – 300	Multivitamin
Vitamin C – 500	Pycnogenol – 100
Ginkgo Biloba	Inositol – 3000 mg
Mega Biotin – 7500 mcg	Alpha-lipoic acid
Sphingolin	Evening of Primrose oil
Magnesium Oxide	L-Carnitine
Coenzyme Q10	

In addition to the above vitamins, I had shots of Calcium EAP twice a week for about three months.

During this period from '94 to '95, my ALS symptoms were rather stable. I simply was not getting any worse. My right arm was partially paralyzed. My right ankle was stiff. Other than that, I was quite normal. I could walk all right except for the arthritis in my left hip. That caused me to use a cane. Talking, breathing, swallowing, and everything else were quite normal. I did not appreciate the fact that I was stable and not getting worse. Actually, that was quite an accomplishment, but I just did not realize it then. In retrospect, I should have realized that my condition had stabilized. However, I wasn't happy with just staying the same. I wanted improvement. When I didn't improve, I began to shortcut my vitamin regimen. In July of '95, my left hip got so bad with arthritis I had to have a full hip replacement. Now, here's where I find fault with another MD. I asked the doctor before the surgery if any of this would affect my ALS condition. He just shrugged it off and said we're only concerned with you living through the surgery. "Well, OK, you're the doctor." I never want to say that again. I should not have trusted him; I should have pursued that much further. Immediately following the hip replacement in July of '95, my ALS symptoms worsened. Up to that time, I only had limited motion in my right hand and arm and in my right foot. After the surgery, it moved into my left arm and left leg and my right leg got worse. They had given me morphine for pain in the hospital. They had also given me morphine to take home. I was taking the morphine off and on and after some time I realized that when I took the morphine, I was much weaker for one or two days afterwards. I immediately quit using the morphine and I quit having the relapses.

Although my ALS condition got a lot worse following the surgery, it remained stable from then on through '96. When I was diagnosed in '91, the doctor said I had a motor neuron problem, but he didn't call it ALS. I know now that he thought it was ALS but couldn't tell me that. Since then, there have been three situations involving three different doctors who were reluctant to tell me I had ALS. They may not realize it, but I think they do you an injustice by *not* telling you. My alternative treatment doctor never told me I had ALS. However, in a discussion with one of his nurses, she told me I had ALS. Now, how do you like that? The nurse tells you more than the doctor. Well, that's not the first time that happened.

My wife, Glenna, seeing my condition worsen following the '95 surgery, finally convinced me to go for further diagnosis. I agreed. We considered all the major hospitals like UCLA, Scripps, and Loma Linda. We settled on Loma Linda. We first visited an MS specialist. After a very thorough physical exam, he referred me to the ALS specialist. The ALS doctor gave me an EMG, spinal tap, and bone marrow biopsy. All these tests were negative for other diseases. Therefore, the conclusion is ALS.

Following these tests, I immediately began to deteriorate. My entire body got weaker. I began to choke on my food. My speech became slurred. In a very short time, I lost 15 pounds. That's a lot for my body weight. I started at 155 pounds.

These worsening symptoms and the ALS diagnosis are what really motivated me. I had a tremendous fear of ending up totally paralyzed, lying flat on my back, with nothing to do but think. That fear made me finally decide to go all out to beat this nightmare. That meant giving up my daily ration of Coors beer that I had enjoyed for around 40 years. It also meant no coffee, no ice cream and on and on; but I just had to do it. I decided to follow the advice given earlier by my "alternative treatment" doctor. That is, make your body as pure and pristine as possible! In other words, avoid ALL toxins. I immediately put together what I will call my program. I was so convinced that my program would work that I wanted to write an article for the *"ALS Digest."* That's the e-mail newsletter that is published two or three times a week and e-mailed to over 5100+ PALS worldwide. I really wanted to share my ideas with the ALS world. However, my better judgement prevailed. I thought I had better wait until I've proven it before I write. I waited one year and after a great deal of improvement, I wrote my first article for the *"ALS Digest."*

Now, let's get back to reviewing my program. We have already discussed PMA, prayer, and belief. As you will recall, my program has three parts or three steps:

Step 1 – Avoid all toxins.
Step 2 – Take all reasonable treatments to remove toxins from the body.
Step 3 – Provide the body with proper diet and dietary supplements.

Let me clarify something here; something I have learned only recently. I believe we should look at the treatment of ALS as being in two phases.

PHASE ONE – The object of Phase One is to *stop the progress of ALS.*

PHASE TWO – The object of Phase Two is to *restore the body* to its former condition.

Here is the basic idea in recognizing two phases. If your home was on fire, you would not start rebuilding your home until you first put out the fire. The same thing applies to treating your ALS condition. You must emphasize Phase One treatments before you go too far with Phase Two treatments. For example: Any form of detoxification is a Phase One treatment. The controversial stem cell treatment is obviously a Phase Two treatment. It restores brain cells but does nothing to put out the fire. I believe you should know your objective before starting any treatment.

There are many electrical treatments available. I believe in the possible benefits from electromagnetic treatments such as the Wet Cell Battery treatment. However, I believe that is a Phase Two treatment. Not that you couldn't do it in Phase One, but if you have limited financial resources and time, you should first spend it on Phase One treatments. Additionally, a Phase Two treatment might result in some improvement even though you have not eliminated the toxin causing your problem. In other words, it might give you a false reading. I believe it is absolutely critical to first stop the progress of ALS and that can only be done permanently by detoxifying the body.

I have not tried the Wet Cell Treatment but I think it has merit. It was recommended in the readings of Edgar Cayce. He was a remarkable man and had an unusual gift for healing. If you are interested in the Wet Cell Treatment, call Baar Products Inc:

(800) 269-2502 or e-mail *bbaar@baar.com.*

There is a lot of attention right now being focused on stem cell research. This could be a major breakthrough. However, I think it is a Phase Two treatment, not Phase One. Replacement of stem cells treats the symptom but not the cause.

There is another Phase Two treatment that I must mention: Human Growth Hormone Replacement. This is another one that I have not tried because it is very expensive. However, if I could afford it, I would do it.

Update – March 2004

Well, guess what? I began HGH injections a year and a half ago. I believe HGH is helping me. More on this later.

The three-part program discussed earlier in this chapter will be reviewed in more detail in the next three chapters.

It should be noted that this is simply a health improvement program. We want to do everything possible to help the body help itself. This program, or a similar one, could be used to improve one's health regardless of what health problem may exist. This is a full body treatment program. You're treating the mind, heart, and body. It is not a band-aid treatment. It is not a "treat the symptom" approach. There is no doubt in my mind but what my program is responsible for me being alive today. It also means I will probably live many more years. Let me remind you that I am not a doctor and I am not recommending any treatment for you. My program works for me. However, I recommend that you find a health practitioner, preferably a medical doctor, who deals with alternative treatments. You should not follow my program; rather use it as a guide and under the direction of a professional healthcare person.

CHAPTER 7

AVOID ALL TOXINS

Part One of My Program

This chapter on avoiding toxins and the next one on detox are the two most important. I'm really not sure which one should come first but since amalgam removal is part of avoiding toxins I will start with that one. The main reason for this is that amalgam removal is the first thing you should do in avoiding toxins and amalgam removal should take place **before** any serious detox treatment such as chelation. If I had any dental amalgams containing mercury, I would have them removed at once. You must find a dentist who is experienced in amalgam removal and will take all the necessary precautions during removal. You may want to order the information kit from DAMS as previously discussed. You should be thoroughly acquainted with the correct procedures and be sure to select a dentist who will follow them.

Avoiding toxins is a big order. There are so many toxins in our food and environment it's probably safe to say that you can't do this 100%. My grandma would get after me for saying, "can't." Oh well, we have to do our best, but be realistic and settle for 99%. Toxins are in the air, the water, and the food we eat.

If you live where the air is pure and clean, you are indeed fortunate. I previously lived in Orange County (that's where Disneyland is), which is adjacent to Los Angeles, California. L.A. is Smog City. Orange County is not much better. I was fortunate in a way that when I got ALS, I was near retirement. I was able to retire and move to Desert Hot Springs in the California desert where the air is reasonably clean.

Water often contains many toxins. Tap water in almost all areas of the U.S. should be avoided for drinking and cooking purposes. Desert Hot Springs has, from what I've read, the purest water of anyplace in the U.S. It is so pure they do not have to add chlorine. I even had the water tested for heavy metals namely aluminum, arsenic, lead and mercury. They all four were below reportable limits. A lot of people drink tap water even though they know chlorine is in it. They must think chlorine is all right. However, it is *not all right.* It is toxic. The bleach you put in your washing machine to brighten your clothes is the same thing as chlorine. Would you drink a glass of that bleach? Well, if you drink tap water, you're already drinking bleach.

To illustrate the harmful effects of chlorine in the tap water, let me tell you a story about my fishpond. I built a waterfall and large fishpond in each of the last five homes I have lived in. In order to clean the fishpond, I used to remove the fish and put them in a large plastic trash barrel, fill it with fresh tap water, and leave the hose in it providing a supply of fresh water. Three times, and at two different locations, I killed all my Koi fish doing this. I eventually learned (I guess I'm a slow learner) that the fresh water contained so much chlorine it was killing the fish. The last time this happened was at my home in Wildomar, California where we had a swimming pool. I had the test kit for the swimming pool, which gave me the necessary items to test water for chlorine content. I tested the tap water and you won't want to believe this. The tap water had the perfect amount of chlorine that you should have in your swimming pool. When I say perfect, I mean perfect. Now let me ask you. Would you want to drink the water in your pool, which you know contains chlorine; of course not. However, you may be drinking water from your tap that is the same as your swimming pool water.

Actually, chlorine is not the only bad toxin that may be in your tap water. Fluoride has been added to the tap water in many cities within the USA. **Fluoride is toxic.** It is made using the waste material from chemical plants. Can you believe that? There may be many others such as mercury, lead, arsenic, and other heavy metals that may cause even more harm. Our water systems are being polluted with many different toxins in all parts of our country.

Okay, we all must agree that tap water needs to be avoided, so let's buy some bottled water at the supermarket or obtain bottled water from some company who delivers it to your home. Well from what I have read, that might not be the answer either. I've read that much of the bottled water is not pure and the plastic container may even be made of carcinogenic material. Well what do we do?

If you don't have a source of quality water, like we have in Desert Hot Springs, then I think your best bet is distilled water in glass containers for your drinking. Better yet, I would buy the best water filter money can buy; one that would filter the water for your entire home.

So much for the air and water, let's talk about food. Amalgams are a major source of toxins and you use them to chew your food. We have already discussed amalgams, but let me restate here that they need to be eliminated.

The best way to avoid as many toxins as possible is to eat only *fresh* food: *fresh* vegetables, *fresh* fruit, *fresh* nuts, etc. You will find that almost all foods that have been processed, frozen, or packaged contain some toxic preservative or taste enhancer. Here again, you need the help of a nutritionist. The fresh food should be **organically grown** to avoid pesticides and herbicides, which, of course, are toxic. I have found it difficult to obtain high quality organically grown produce in my area. Therefore, I have been forced to buy produce from the local market. The next best thing is to thoroughly wash and soak your produce in a product called "Healthy Harvest Fruit & Vegetable Rinse." This is the safe way to remove pesticides, chemical residues, wax, dirt and bacteria from your fresh produce. At least that is what the label says. We use it and it seems to work quite well.

Before we get into some details on diet, let's discuss diet in general. Let me first ask you a question. If you bought a new, expensive automobile and the dealer told you that the automobile was designed for a certain type of gasoline, would you follow his instructions or would you try to operate it by using kerosene because kerosene is cheaper. Well, I feel quite certain that you would not run your car on kerosene for any reason. However, we all do something quite different when it comes to fuel for our body. For thousands of years, our ancestors ate food that was naturally grown. They ate it fresh from the tree or vine. They did not have supermarkets, refrigerators, or freezers. You might say, therefore, our bodies were designed to be fueled by that same diet. If your car had problems and you told your mechanic that you are running it on kerosene, he would tell you immediately to run it on the fuel for which it was designed. Doesn't it stand to reason that we should do the same thing with our bodies? In other words, when we get sick, shouldn't we first consider going back to a basic diet of fresh, raw food to restore our health?

In the event that some of you may "pooh-pooh" what I'm saying about the safety of food in the markets, let me stir you up a little. In the local paper on August 1, 1999, there was an article about genetically altered food. According to this article, 60% of food in the market already contains some biotech-made ingredient. Now I for one don't like this. Why? Because it *ain't* natural. Don't fool with Mother Nature is one of my beliefs. They have already developed a vegetable plant that excretes a substance that is toxic to insects. Well, that's just great, but when we eat the vegetable, don't we then eat the toxin too?

There's another one that was in the paper August 9, 1999. Scientists now believe that the "mad cow disease" in England a few years ago was caused by a scientific experiment that went bad. This blunder cost England 6.4 billion dollars and already killed 43 people with many more to come. The experts say that they were taking hormones from the brains of dead animals and injecting them into cows in order to create a stronger breed of cattle. Here again, they're fooling around with Mother Nature and I don't like it! However, it is proof again that we cannot trust the food in the market to be safe.

Now, back to my diet. This kind of a diet means you must eliminate some things you may really like. Here are just a few examples of what I eliminated from my diet:

> Coffee (including decaf) and tea (other than herbal tea or
> green tea)
> Ice cream

Animal products including meat and dairy products like milk.
I did not eliminate butter because I just can't live
without it and I believe margarine is worse than butter.
Canned goods
Soft drinks
Alcoholic beverages
Sugar (Also avoid foods that contain sugar)
Don't use Aspartame (NutraSweet).

A great sugar substitute is Stevia Extract. Get it at
your health food store. It is expensive, but a little bit
goes a long way. Three or four drops on a bowl of cold
cereal and milk (rice milk) are plenty.

Another great sugar substitute is Nature's Taste
granular dietary supplement by Amazon Natural
Treasures, 4011 W. Oquendo Rd., #C, Las Vegas, Nevada
89118.

Honey is also a great substitute for sugar
particularly in hot beverages.

Salt and black pepper (Cayenne pepper may be OK)

Salt is a poison. Eat enough of it and it can kill you.
However, the little bit of salt you may sprinkle on your
eggs is not the problem. The real intake of salt occurs
when you eat bacon, sausage, lunchmeat like bologna,
olives and pickles. These food items are saturated with
salt. At the start of my program, I eliminated salt 100%.
However, after a year of eating food cooked with no salt,
I couldn't stand it anymore. I've added salt (sea salt) to
our cooking but use no salt otherwise. If you include any
salt in your diet, I would recommend sea salt that is
available at your health food store.

These are just some examples of items that you may want to
eliminate from your diet. I think the most important items on this list
are sugar, MSG, and Aspartame. They should be avoided like the plague.
More on MSG later. Again, work with a nutritionist.

Most nutritionists will recommend that you avoid all dairy products and wheat products. The reason is many people have allergic reactions to wheat and dairy products. My theory is that if some people are allergic to certain foods, then they may not be good for any of us. Therefore, why take a chance? Eliminate it from your diet.

Milk

Here's another reason you may want to avoid milk.

A recent investigation found that PALS have a greater exposure to lead and mercury and drink more milk than other control patients. The obvious conclusion is there is a relationship between lead, mercury and excessive milk ingestion and ALS. Excessive milk ingestion was indicated to be three or more glasses a day. Coincidentally, from age 0 to 35, I drank at least one glass of milk with every meal or three glasses a day. That's a pretty interesting coincidence, wouldn't you say?

Additionally, do not cook or prepare foods in aluminum cookware or aluminum foil. The best cooking utensil is one made of stainless steel or glass.

If you cover food to be heated or cooked in a microwave, do not use plastic. If you must use plastic, do not let it touch the food. Of course you can't use metal in the microwave, so glass is the best container to use.

The following is an example of what you can eat and be reasonably safe. This is what I have been eating for seven years now with good results.

Breakfast

Two eggs (see note below) fried in butter, scrambled or poached (I know I said no dairy products, but I can't live without a little butter).

OR

Six-grain cereal which includes oatmeal. You buy this fresh from the health food store. No milk. In the beginning, I used Rice Dream milk, which is a non-dairy product available in health food stores. Then, I learned that rice was acidic and soy milk is alkaline. Therefore, if you want to correct your pH to more alkaline, then soy milk would be better.

OR

Bananas sliced on cold cereal but only a cereal sold at the health food store with no preservatives. Again, use rice or soy milk. *NOTE:* I had been eating bananas all along until recently. See my special note below on bananas.

A special note on bananas

Bananas – current update

I have to laugh when I tell you this story about bananas. You may find some humor in it too. I think I'm doing everything right and avoiding toxins, when suddenly I learned about another one I must avoid.

In the book on chelation that will be discussed in the next chapter, there's a short discussion on pesticides. According to the book, there are many pesticides that are now illegal to use here in the U.S.A. Therefore, the producers of these banned pesticides sell them to other countries. The other countries use these pesticides on their crops, such as bananas, and then sell their crops to the U.S.A.

Do you see the humor in that?

I believe the problem with these illegal pesticides is that they do not dissipate. They get into the soil and the roots of the plant. Then they are absorbed in the plant and ultimately the fruit of the plant.

You know that I've said before that if there's any chance that something will adversely affect my health, I will avoid it. I thought that bananas in the supermarket were relatively safe. However, I now prefer to buy my organic bananas at the health food store.

A special note on eggs

I know I mentioned earlier to avoid all animal products. However, I consider eggs and butter as an exception to that rule. Right or wrong, I eat eggs. It is my personal belief that eggs have been given a bum rap. Eggs are a near perfect whole food and relatively uncontaminated by food additives. It is preferable to use eggs from free-range chickens. One reason they tell us to not eat eggs is that you will develop high cholesterol and high blood pressure. I am 72 years old in the year 2001 and I eat eggs damned near everyday. I was recently tested for cholesterol and it is in the "perfect" range. Also my blood pressure is consistently around 110/70. That is the typical blood pressure for a twenty-year-old. How about that sports fans?!

Lunch

Lunch begins with a glass of "Eric's Veggie Delight." Doesn't that just make your mouth water?

Glenna, my wife and caregiver, spends about an hour of everyday preparing this tasty cocktail. You must have a vegetable juicer. Buy a good one with mostly stainless steel parts and less plastic. We use a variety of vegetables and fruits, but most often apple, carrots, celery, and beets. I throw in one clove of raw garlic for my arthritis. You can counteract the ill affects of the garlic with a small sprig of parsley. Glenna then transfers this juice to the blender, adds all my vitamins and food supplements, and blends it all together. No, don't just throw your tablets and capsules in the blender. The tablets must be crushed into a powder first. We use a "pestle and mortar" to grind them to a fine powder. You pull the capsules apart and dump the contents in the blender and discard the shell. Gel caps, like Vitamin E, have to be taken separately. Some vitamins, like Vitamin A, you can get in oil form. Just pour them in the blender.

Glenna makes a 12-ounce drink that we split in half, providing a six-ounce "luscious cocktail" for lunch and another six-ounce drink for dinner. This is a rich diet and can sometimes cause diarrhea. I use a product called Original Papaya Enzymes made by American Health and available from the health food store. These are chewable tablets. If you can't chew them, you could easily crush them and mix them with a liquid. They taste great. These enzyme tablets are primarily an aid to digestion. They can be used for indigestion or to prevent indigestion, if taken at the end of a meal. I discovered, quite accidentally, that they seem to help me avoid diarrhea. I take two, three or four with every meal as needed. In my humble opinion, Alka-Seltzer, Bromo-Seltzer and all the others would be out of business if everyone knew about these enzymes (no I don't sell them). There are a few fantastic inventions in the world today and my favorites are Band-Aids, Kleenex, and ChapStick. In my book, these are everyday essentials. These enzyme tablets rank right up there with them.

In addition to my veggie cocktail for lunch, I eat a banana quite often. Occasionally I have a bowl of rice (natural brown rice from the health food store only), or a fried egg sandwich on rye (no wheat bread) or some fresh fruit.

I don't eat too much fresh fruit, other than bananas or apples, because of my tendency toward diarrhea. Also, one of my doctors said I should avoid sugar including fresh fruit, other than apples and bananas.

Dinner

Dinner begins with the second veggie cocktail of the day. Most often that's followed by a large plate of *steamed* vegetables; not boiled or fried. Steaming is the best way to prepare your veggies for flavor and retention of vitamins and nutrients. Get yourself a stainless steel pot and insert a stainless steel steam basket. Place the veggies in the basket. It holds them up above the boiling water. We cook all the following vegetables in one pot. If you cut them into small pieces about the same size, they will all cook within 30 minutes; including potatoes. We usually use white potatoes, yams, cauliflower, broccoli, green beans, turnips, brussels sprouts, asparagus and all kinds of squash.

The large leaf vegetables like spinach, beet tops, kale, Swiss chard and rapini are cooked separately in a boiling pot. You can't very well steam them. I have a bowl of these boiled greens, in addition to steamed veggies, two or three times a week. This would be a tasteless mess without adding onions and garlic. Sauté the onions and garlic in butter, then add water and bring to a boil. Add the cleaned and cut greens to the boiling water. Boil until fully cooked. This comes out quite flavorful. I eat my greens with a small amount of vinegar added at the table. Use unfiltered apple cider vinegar purchased at the health food store.

Meat or Beef

Occasionally we supplement the veggie meal with a bowl of natural brown rice or some meat. However, here is a word of caution on meat. Man is an omnivorous animal. He is neither carnivorous nor vegetarian. Man has been eating both vegetables *and* meat for thousands of years. We should not suddenly become a vegetarian, nor should we eat meat exclusively. We must have both protein and veggies. Many people, who do eat both meat and veggies, still get it wrong. Most people eat more meat and fewer veggies. It should be the other way around. We need a lot of veggies.

I communicated with a lady PALS who had ALS over 20 years and was getting along quite well. I pay attention to people like this, to see what I can learn. She felt that protein was bad for her and she was a vegetarian. She said that every time she added protein to her diet, it made her worse. This is, of course, very controversial. My conclusion, right or wrong, is that we need some protein but not a lot. In the first year of my program, I did not eat any meat. I included a small amount of protein powder in my daily drink. Once I had reversed my ALS symptoms, I began to add meat occasionally.

Dioxin has been in the news a lot lately. It is a known cancer-causing toxin. Recent studies show that it may be ten times more toxic than previously thought. The news announcements said it occurred primarily in meat and dairy products and they recommended avoiding them as much as possible.

Most beef is full of hormones, preservatives, tenderizers and who knows what else. You may want to check with your local meat markets and find one which sells organically raised beef. It may be more expensive but it may also taste better. An interesting side note is that for the last ten years or more, prior to my program, I was developing a dislike for beef. It just did not taste the same to me as it did years ago.

Well, let me tell you that the organically raised beef that we buy has the same flavor that I remember from the past.

Chicken

I rarely eat chicken. If I do, it is chicken that is organically raised and the skin is removed before it is cooked. According to an article in *"The Los Angeles Times,"* on March 2, 2002, Russia will ban imports of U.S. poultry as of March 10, 2002. Their concern was that the chlorine-based disinfectants used by producers may cause cancer. Additionally, Russia requested a list of drugs and hormones added to the chicken feed and the U.S. failed to respond. Now that friend is enough to make me not eat chicken unless organically raised.

Lamb

Lamb is probably no better than any other meat, but I eat it anyway because lamb is my favorite meat. If I could find organically raised lamb, I would certainly prefer that. I only eat lamb about once a week or less.

Fish

What about fish? Well, when I first started my program, I ate a lot of fish because I was avoiding beef and other meat. However, since then, I have learned more and more about fish containing mercury. Sometime ago, there was a discussion on TV about some fish containing high levels of mercury. Additionally, I have read several articles in our local newspaper about fish and mercury. One article was about two rivers in the High Sierra mountain range of central California. This is the old Gold Rush area and they used mercury to separate gold from the ore. The mercury is still polluting our rivers and the fish in them. In the newspaper article, they were considering posting mercury warnings on the rivers. The other article discussed the fact that about 60,000 babies are born each year in the U.S. and they face serious threat of neurological damage because their mothers eat fish contaminated with mercury. They seem to think that babies are the only ones faced with a problem from mercury. Well, I think that's really dumb. Maybe I'm the only one, but I don't eat fish anymore except those that I've caught in the eastern Sierras, which I think, are relatively free of mercury.

In a recent article in March 2004, the FDA warned against pregnant women eating too much fish. They caution against eating certain fish more than once a week such as tuna, albacore, swordfish and salmon (most salmon available today is **farmed** salmon) and that should be avoided. **Wild** salmon may be OK. Since the big fish eat the little fish, the fish that are further up the food chain have a higher amount of mercury.

In my opinion, the FDA is overly political. If it were up to me, I would recommend eating no fish because there's **no safe amount of mercury for your body.**

Do you think we are doing all we can to avoid toxins? Not on your life; there is much more. I can't cover it all, but I will list all the things I have done to avoid toxins:

Insecticides

We don't ever use ant spray or other insecticides in the house. We don't even store them in the house. You do not want to breathe any vapor from them.

Pet Flea Collars

The flea collars that we used for years on both our cat and our dog were removed and discarded. Fortunately, we live in the dry desert and we learned that we don't have fleas here. Isn't that great!

Gasoline

The fumes in the gasoline station are toxic and should be avoided. My wife pumps the gas while I remain in the car with all of the windows up. Some peach of a wife, huh?

Self-Cleaning Ovens

You do not want to be anywhere in the house when you're in the process of cleaning the self-cleaning oven. The vapors are highly toxic.

Toothpaste

One day I was reading the label on my normal toothpaste. It said, "If you swallow more toothpaste than the amount you use to brush with, contact your Poison Control Center or see your doctor at once." I said earlier that I'm not a fast learner. However, that told me right away that the toothpaste I was using was toxic. Since it is toxic, I don't even want it in my mouth for a minute. For a while I brushed with baking soda and salt. That's what everyone used before toothpaste was invented. Then I discovered a natural toothpaste at the health food store called Weleda. It is a salt toothpaste with baking soda and is detergent free. I use this exclusively now and it works just fine.

Ceramic or Pottery Dishes, Cups & Bowls

Many ceramic and pottery dishes are made with lead. Lead is a toxin and lead can get into the food you eat from your ceramic dishes, cups and bowls. You want to be sure that none of your dishes are contaminating your food with lead. You can even test your dishes with a kit from Frandon Enterprises Inc., 511 North 48th Street, Seattle, Washington 98103.

Drugs

Did you ever wonder why prescription drugs require a prescription? The answer is simple: they are **dangerous**.

Many if not most prescription drugs are toxic to your system. In spite of that, medical doctors give out prescriptions like candy. Most drugs have bad side effects because of their toxicity. If you don't believe this, let me support it with some figures.

I've read two different articles stating that over 100,000 people die annually in the U.S. from prescription drugs. That does not count overdoses or pharmacist errors. Additionally, it only includes those that occur in the hospital. Those that occur outside hospitals go unrecorded many times. A recent newspaper article quoted an HMO executive as saying the figure was more like 180,000 a year.

100,000 people every year is a lot. To put that in better perspective, legal prescription drugs are the fourth leading cause of death in the U.S.

A good example of this is the drugs used to treat arthritis. The effect of the arthritis drug is limited to relieving pain primarily. They offer no cure or even improvement in the arthritic condition. The FDA estimates that there are 200,000 cases of gastrointestinal bleeding that occur each year from the use of these drugs. Additionally, and more importantly, there are between 10,000 and 20,000 patients who *die* from these drugs. Now, that's only one example. There are many more. Another example is drugs to treat cholesterol. Have you ever heard the expression "What fools these mortals be?" Well, the drug companies are really making fools of us on these cholesterol drugs and here is why I say that.

1. First of all, there is no clear-cut evidence that high cholesterol *alone* has any direct relationship to a higher death rate. The situation is much more complex. I have read that it is much more important to lower your triglycerides than your cholesterol. Additionally, there is good cholesterol or HDL and there is bad cholesterol LDL. You really want to take a supplement that will lower the LDL and raise the HDL. Several years ago I read about a study on cholesterol. They divided a controlled group into two. They fed one group a high cholesterol diet and the other group a low cholesterol diet. The high cholesterol group had a higher fatality rate from heart attacks. However, the overall death rate of both groups was normal. Why? The low cholesterol group had a higher fatality rate from cancer. You see cholesterol is a life-giving element. If you have none of it, you will die.

2. The body produces 80% of your cholesterol.
3. There are many natural foods and supplements that can reduce your cholesterol *and* that are very safe. A few examples are garlic, olive oil, avocados, onions, niacin, lecithin, chromium, and zinc. Of all these, lecithin is my favorite. Lecithin occurs naturally in eggs. That's why if you eat eggs you won't necessarily have high cholesterol. The same is true of raw milk. Raw milk is milk taken directly from the cow: totally natural. Raw milk contains lecithin and lecithin is destroyed in the process of pasteurizing and homogenizing of the milk. A study of a group of people who were fed one pint of raw milk daily showed no signs of higher cholesterol and no higher fatality rate than normal.
4. Additionally, a lower intake of all fats will reduce your cholesterol.

In my humble opinion, it is absolutely criminal for anyone to prescribe a cholesterol reducing drug without first trying all the natural treatments. Of course we must realize that most people don't want to do that. They want a pill, so their doctor gives them one.

Let's talk about the time the doctor had me take Flagyl four separate times. They had me take Flagyl again and again without any concern about side effects or any forethought about what they were doing. I read somewhere that to continue doing the same exact thing, and expecting different results, is a mild form of insanity. I couldn't agree more. Prior to the *second* dose of Flagyl, I *suggested* to my doctor that we do something different. Prior to the *third* time, I *begged* him to do something different. The *fourth* time I *insisted* that we do something different and we did; and I was finally cured. However, on the second and third time, the doctor said, "Oh, we'll just try it again." They never, ever considered doing anything differently nor did they do any research. They just gave me another prescription for Flagyl. It's a wonder they didn't kill me with Flagyl.

When it comes to prescription drugs other than antibiotics, I think we're going down the wrong road. We're being led down the road by *money* followed close behind by the drug companies. The drug companies are followed by the AMA. This is a sad parade. *Remember this; you can make more money by treating an illness than you can by curing an illness.* Drugs, other than antibiotics, do not cure because they don't treat the *cause* of the illness. They only treat the symptom. For the last fifty years, the drug companies have been the number one money making industry in the stock market.

OK, drugs are toxic; I hope you agree. Everyone should minimize the use of drugs. This is extremely important for PALS. I already told you about the bad effect I had from morphine. There are many natural substances that do not have bad side effects that should be considered first. In Germany, for example, medical doctors prescribe St. John's Wort 70% of the time for depression. I don't know what percent in the U.S., but I'm sure it's a long way from 70%.

Incidentally, Valium seems to not be detrimental, but can be habit forming. It is the only drug I have taken in the last few years and then I only took one pill prior to some dental work. My ALS doctor approved it. Oops, I forgot one other drug. Since I had my hip replacement surgeries, the doctor insists that I take an antibiotic an hour before any dental work. You should check with your ALS doctor before taking any drug or medication.

Miscellaneous Sprays and Vapors

You obviously want to avoid all industrial vapors and spray paints, etc. However, what about hair spray for example? That certainly seems harmless enough. Well, it isn't. Read the label and you'll see. Almost everything in a spray can is suspect of being toxic. I prefer not to be in the same room when someone is using hair spray, deodorant spray, finger nail polish or anything else of that nature. Also, household cleansers are almost all toxic and should be avoided. You can substitute many non-toxic natural cleaning agents such as lemon juice, baking soda, vinegar, etc. You can clean your windows by spraying them with club soda and wipe them down. Use olive oil and lemon juice for furniture polish.

Most perfumes are toxic and even perfumed candles can be toxic.

Air

Yes, I'm talking about the air you breathe. Most people know that the air is highly polluted around cities and industrial plants. If you live in an area like that, you may not be able to avoid polluted air. However, you may not be able to beat ALS either because of it. We know from studies that polluted air can cause cancer. Additionally, recent studies involving several U.S. cities and several cities in foreign countries have shown smog to be harmful to babies and fetuses. The problems cited included low birth weight, premature birth, stillborn, and infant deaths. Now if smog can hurt even a fetus growing in the mother's womb, then it must be harmful to all of us.

Well, so much for the outdoor air, but what about the air inside your home? You may find it hard to believe, but the indoor air is even worse. Articles I have read say that indoor air in the average home is polluted three times more than the outdoor air. One article even said it could be five times more polluted. There are so many different air-polluting toxins that you may not be able to eliminate them all. Perhaps one should eliminate as many as possible and then buy an air purifier. I am considering buying one now.

Update – March 2004

We now have four Ionic Breeze air purifiers in our home and we love them. More on that later.

Remember that my theory is that when you have ALS, you have weak tissue and your body is more susceptible to harm by all toxins including the polluted air you breathe. You must avoid this if at all possible. It is my belief that unless you eliminate your exposure to *all* toxins you may never win the battle.

Other Toxins

Avoid polyester clothing. They contain toxic chemicals including formaldehyde.

Avoid wearing clothing that has been dry cleaned. Again, toxic chemicals are used.

Wash all new clothing before wearing for the same reason.

Don't use fabric softeners including dryer sheets. We use ¼ cup distilled white vinegar and add to the rinse cycle.

Use non-scented toilet tissue without color print.

Mothballs should be thrown out and not used anywhere in your home.

Avoid cigarette smoke. Second-hand smoke is toxic.

"Eric, aren't you being a little paranoid about this toxic stuff?" Well, maybe. However when your life is at stake, can you be too cautious? You can't afford not to be cautious. If there is one chance in a thousand that something could be harmful to you, why take the chance, unless there is some other giant benefit. Did you read that story in the newspaper about the kid who died from spraying his body with underarm deodorant? No, I'm not kidding. Apparently he thought if one was good, two is better! If spraying the underarm was good, then spraying his whole body was better. Well, so much for that rule. I don't know if he died from toxins in the deodorant or from the deodorant plugging up all his pores so the body couldn't breathe. The newspaper article did not explain that. However, it doesn't matter to me. Either way, if a lot is bad, then a little can't be good, for whatever reason. Stay close to nature.

Here is another story on vapors that will fog your brain. In a recent letter to Dear Abby, the writer explained the death of her 6'1" 190 lb. 16-year-old son. He died after sniffing a tissue roll stuffed with paper soaked with deodorant spray. Does that surprise you? It does me too, but again it proves how toxic some of these chemicals are that are in the items we use everyday.

Over the last seven years that I have been on my program, I have been generally improving. However, occasionally I have a relapse. That is a situation where I suddenly get weaker all over my body and the weakness lasts about 36 hours. Then, I'm back to where I was before the relapse. In every case, I can trace the cause to a toxin. Usually, it's something in the food such as MSG. You see, I'm human like anyone else, and I get damned tired of my strict diet and occasionally try something I shouldn't. Every time I'm forced back on my original program. I am convinced that if I did not stay on my strict diet I would not continue to improve.

We've spent a lot of time talking about toxins and yet we haven't defined toxin. Just to be sure that we all understand, let's elaborate some. Toxin means poison. Poison means toxin. The dictionary defines both as something that will kill or injure. In actual use, I think poison is more associated with killing and a toxin is associated more with damage or injury.

The human body is truly remarkable. It can withstand small amounts of most any poison or toxin. However, larger doses can be fatal. Small doses, repeated over a long period of time, can be fatal also. The body can only stand so much. We tend to overlook this when handling toxins such as insecticides and others that we have discussed. However, as an ALS patient, you can no longer afford the risk.

We've covered a lot of toxins, which are in our air, water, and food, but not all of them. Good grief, can there be more? You bet, and some of the worse are yet to come.

We're now going to discuss a different kind of toxin: *excitotoxins*. These are toxins that destroy or damage brain and nerve cells by over-stimulation.

MSG

Monosodium Glutamate (MSG) is one such *excitotoxin*. MSG is a taste enhancer. It is a food additive used by almost all the food companies today.

Here's how it works. The motor neuron brain cells are activated by glutamate. MSG is a form of glutamate. A little bit of glutamate has to be in your system in order for these brain cells to function. However, an excess amount of glutamate can burn out these motor neuron brain cells. We might compare this to the light bulb and electricity. As long as the light bulb receives a measured and controlled amount of electricity, it will burn for months and months. However, if the electricity is increased suddenly, the bulb burns out in a split second. I'm hardly a specialist in this area but that's what I've read. If you question this, or anything I'm about to say regarding MSG, please read the books first. I have read two books about MSG, both written by medical doctors, each of whom accumulated a ton of information about MSG. The books are:

"*Excitotoxins, The Taste That Kills*" by R.L. Blaylock, MD

"*In Bad Taste, The MSG Syndrome*" by George Schwartz, MD

The authors of these two books are very convincing about the health hazard that exists from overuse of MSG. They also discuss aspartame (NutraSweet) as an equally toxic ingredient. They make a pretty good argument in favor of eliminating both of them from our diets. However, that is very difficult to do unless you follow a diet similar to the one we've already discussed. I tell you this in an effort to give you more cause to follow that kind of a program.

The National Institute of Occupational Safety & Health of the Department of Health & Human Services "*Hazardous Desk Reference*" gives MSG the worst possible toxicity rating (HR3) while the FDA rates it "GRAS," generally regarded as safe!

Well, why the conflict? I can't make accusations, but we all know that "money talks."

Now, let's look at some new information on MSG. The following is a quote from the National Organization Mobilized to Stop Glutamate (NOMSG). This organization has since ceased to exist. I would hazard a guess that they were put out of business somehow by the MSG industry.

* * *

"MSG is a Drug & Neurotransmitter

The ever-expanding use of MSG causes great concern in the medical profession because it stimulates brain cell activity. MSG "tricks" your brain into thinking the food you are eating tastes good. Manufacturers can use inferior ingredients and thus make the product seem tastier. Inferior products and higher profits prevail at the expense of consumer health. MSG intolerance is not an allergic reaction, but a powerful drug reaction.

Common reactions:

Headache, migraine, stomach upset, fatigue, nausea and vomiting, diarrhea, irritable bowel syndrome, asthma attacks, shortness of breath, anxiety or panic attacks, heart palpitations, partial paralysis, "heart attack-like symptoms," balance difficulties, mental confusion, mood swings, depression, behavior disorders (especially in children and teens), allergy-type symptoms, skin rashes, runny nose, bags under the eyes, flushing, mouth lesions, and more.

Hidden sources of MSG:

Definite sources of MSG:

Hydrolyzed Protein
Sodium Caseinate or Calcium Caseinate
Autolyzed Yeast or Yeast Extract
Gelatin

Possible sources of MSG:

Textured Protein
Carrageenan or Vegetable Gum
Seasonings or Spices
Flavorings or Natural Flavorings
Chicken, Beef, Pork, Smoke Flavorings
Bouillon, Broth or Stock
Barley Malt, Malt Extract, Malt Flavoring
Whey Protein, Whey Protein Isolate or Concentrate
Soy Protein, Soy Protein Isolate or Concentrate
Soy Sauce or Extract

MSG in its pure form must be labeled. When it is added as an ingredient of another substance it need not be listed on the label. The earlier these substances appear on a list of ingredients, the more likely they are to contain MSG. We advise avoiding all sources listed above. This list is periodically updated by the networking membership of NOMSG. It is not all inclusive because new labeling deceptions are invented to confound the consumer. We can provide an expanded list for those who are extremely sensitive. We also suggest elimination of aspartame (NutraSweet) and sulfites from the diet."

*   *   *

Reprinted with permission from the National Organization Mobilized to Stop Glutamate (NOMSG).

NOMSG previously published a quarterly newsletter. The "*NOMSG Newsletter*" included several letters in each issue from individuals who suffer health problems from MSG. When I read these letters, it makes me furious with the FDA and our government. It is totally unacceptable to see so many people suffering from a food additive approved by the FDA. There are literally thousands of people right here in the USA who are currently suffering from the effects of MSG. Probably there are many who suffer from it and don't even know that MSG is the source of their health problem. Asthma and migraine headaches have increased over 50% in the last ten or twenty years on a per capita basis. Something has to be causing that. I'm reasonably sure that MSG is the culprit. Again, if you have any doubt about that, please read the two books I previously suggested.

Let me tell you a story about one experience I had with MSG. I have always been health conscious and seldom eat in fast food restaurants. However, one day I was really pressed for time between appointments and I drove in to a fast food restaurant for a quickie lunch. I had one of their hamburgers and a vanilla milk shake. Believe me this was a rarity for me. In spite of that, the very next day I was in the same boat and had the same fast food lunch. Starting the evening after the second lunch, I had what I call a relapse. I used to get these relapses occasionally before I started my program. The relapse consists of overall body weakness and fatigue. They last from 24 to 36 hours.

The next time I visited my "alternative treatment" doctor, I told him about the fast food episode and the subsequent relapse. He had no idea what might have caused it but suggested that maybe the sugar in the milk shakes might have done it. It was about two or three months later I was reading the book by Dr. Schwartz on MSG. In his book, he mentioned that many fast food restaurants use MSG in their hamburger meat. That certainly could explain my relapse. In looking back now, I think it was probably the combination of MSG *and* sugar.

I used to have relapses quite frequently, but since I've been on my program, they are non-existent with the exception of a couple of times. Those two or three times occurred immediately after eating in a restaurant. It is very difficult to avoid MSG when eating in restaurants. You can ask them, and I do, if they use MSG. They will normally tell you they do or don't, and if they do, what foods they put it in. However, even if they say they don't use MSG, you still can't be sure. They may use products that contain MSG and they are simply not aware of it. Remember all of the names previously listed that may indicate MSG.

All of the above has been general information on MSG. Now I would like to give you one person's real life experience so you can really see how serious the MSG threat is to your health. I have read many similar letters previously in the "*NOMSG Newsletter*".

The following is a synopsis of a letter from Mrs. D from Grayslake, Illinois:

> She stated that her eleven-year-old son had been very healthy and had a nearly perfect attendance record in school. That all changed in September of 1997 when her son developed changes in his personality and became depressed. In the summer of the same year, he began having frequent headaches and sleeping much more than normal. He became very sickly and had a constant headache for the five months. She took her son to a medical doctor, neurologist, dentist, chiropractor and optometrist. None of these healthcare professionals were able to help.

> Then Mrs. D discovered the NOMSG home page on
> the Internet. Immediately she removed MSG from her son's
> diet. After four days, all of his symptoms were gone.

This is a great letter, in my opinion, evidencing the hazards of MSG. Make note that this is not an isolated case. There are thousands more.

Aspartame

Aspartame is another excitotoxin and taste enhancer. You'll find it in many prepared foods, particularly in "low fat" foods and "diet" soft drinks.

I have always avoided diet soft drinks because I don't like the flavor. More importantly, I see only fat people drinking "diet" soft drinks. I don't want to be fat, so I don't drink "diet" soft drinks. That's a joke folks; time for a little chuckle.

While we are telling funny stories here, let me tell you another one about 'diet' drinks. I saw this in a cartoon in the newspaper recently. The character in the cartoon is ordering lunch in a fast food restaurant. He orders "a bacon cheese burger, french fries, and a 'diet' coke." If you know anything about nutrition, you must see the humor in that.

And now back to a more serious vein.

Aspartame has three components including two amino acids, phenylalanine and aspartic acid. The third component is methanol. Many people lack the enzyme to properly process phenylalanine. An accumulation of phenylalanine can cause brain damage. Also, people with kidney disease or iron deficiency could be at risk.

Methanol, the third ingredient, is a known poison or toxin. Toxic levels of methanol can cause blindness, brain swelling, inflammation of the pancreas and heart muscle, and more.

There is an accumulation of anecdotal evidence indicating that Aspartame can cause many of the same adverse reactions listed previously under MSG.

Cysteine

This is a third and relatively new excitotoxin. It is a taste enhancer just like the other two. I have read that they are using it in some bread, but that's all I know about it.

A lot of toxins have been discussed. Those are only the ones that I have had experience with and/or read about. There may be many more that I don't know about. You need to be always on the alert. If you insist on continuing to eat or drink processed food, learn to read the labels. Look for the list of ingredients.

Late Date Insert

It has been a year or more since I wrote this portion of the book, but I just had an experience that I must tell you about and it belongs in this chapter. This has to do with avoiding toxins.

It has now been over seven years that I've been on my restricted diet, and it gets quite boring after a while. Three times in the last seven years I have tried to expand my diet to include some things I really like, but every time I meet with disastrous results. Every time I add something to my diet like ice cream, I have what I call a "set back." A set back is when I get weaker and more tired. It lasts only about 24 to 36 hours and then I'm back to normal. Every time this happens, I wonder if it's only my imagination or if I'm really reading it right. Well, this last time something happened that really confirms the fact that something damaging has entered my system. Let me tell you what happened.

One of the nerve tests the doctor gives you has to do with your foot. The doctor will grab your heel in one hand and the ball of your foot in the other and press the ball of the foot upward in a brisk motion. If you have nerve damage, then your foot will pulsate up and down. I ride my electric three-wheel cart around in our mobile home park and the asphalt pavement has cracks that are three or four inches wide. When you hit one, you really know it. I recently got on an ice cream kick and within three days I developed a setback. During this setback period, I was riding my electric cart and hitting the cracks in the pavement and that was causing my feet to pulsate up and down. When this pulsating starts, it is difficult to stop it. So, it becomes very annoying when these cracks in the pavement are 50 feet apart and every time you hit one you have a bouncing leg. Now, guess what happened. I returned to my diet, that is, I quit the ice cream. After about two or three days, I was riding my cart hitting the cracks in the pavement at full speed and no bouncing legs. Wow, what a pleasant improvement.

I began thinking about that and here is my conclusion. There is no doubt in my mind now, that when you have a condition like ALS, you have a weak system and ANY toxin can adversely affect you. I believe that what you eat is important, but what you *avoid eating* is probably more important. I believe my success at beating ALS has more to do with that than one would normally think.

Now here is another one that might surprise you as it did me. This is not about food, but rather what you apply to your skin. I have been on my program of avoiding toxins for seven years but here is one that I overlooked.

Previously, every time I took a shower, I would feel tired and lethargic and very weak for about two or three hours afterwards. I had been using a bar soap that came with a cord attached to it so I could hang it around my neck for obvious reasons. However, it was not a *pure* soap of my choice and had a fragrance. Remember, most perfumes are mildly toxic. I attributed my weakness to the hot water in the shower and completely overlooked the soap. I changed soap about two months ago and have not had the usual weakness as before. Additionally, I do think my general strength is improving at a more rapid rate. I wonder where I would be now if I had discovered the soap problem two years ago. Who knows what long-range effect that may have had on me? I know you may find this one hard to believe, and I find it hard to believe also. However, there was nothing else that I changed recently.

This is just another example of how careful you must be. Remember also, that if you have a condition like ALS, then your body is weak and more susceptible to the ill effects of any and all toxins.

Update – March 2004

Here are two more recent experiences that have proven again that avoiding toxins is critical.

You probably will not believe this one, but I swear this is what happened. Included on my list of supplements you will find DHEA. Initially I was taking a prescription required DHEA. Then, like a dummy, I switched to DHEA which is now available in the health food stores. For good reason, I switched back to prescription DHEA. I noticed the capsules were bright blue and green. I thought for a moment that the coloring could be toxic. On second thought, I figured that because I was only taking two a day that there just could not be enough toxin in there to bother me. Well, I guess I'm not so smart after all because here's what happened. I took the DHEA for about two months until it finally dawned on me that I was losing ground. I thought and thought about all the possibilities of a toxin in my food or anywhere. There was simply nothing new in my diet or anywhere else that I could determine except this change in DHEA. So, I stopped taking it. Alas, I could see a return to an improving condition within a week.

I know it's hard to believe that a small amount of toxin, apparently in the coloring of the capsules, could really have any effect on me, but again that's what happened.

I also learned something new. You can order your prescription drugs in a vegetable capsule and they will be clear or white and not colored.

Now for another one on avoiding toxins. About three months ago I had a bladder infection. My doctor recommended a shot of an antibiotic and some antibiotic pills. I had one shot and then took the pills for ten days. When I first got the bladder infection, it really affected my ALS condition. My muscles just almost shut down and it was very difficult to move around. Within 24 hours of the antibiotic shot, I was back to my normal ability to move about. Now, here is the interesting part. Within another 24 hours I was better than I was before the bladder infection. That is the kind of experience that really gets my attention.

I had a previous bladder infection about a year ago and I had this same experience, but I just ignored it. Now that it happened twice, I thought more about it. To my way of thinking, this experience must prove my theory about toxins having an unusually bad affect on PALS. But there's more to that. The improvement on the second day after the shot must mean that there is another infection in my body that I don't know about. I asked my doctor to let me continue the shots to see what would happen. I took the antibiotic for four weeks. I really believe that my condition improved as a result. I'm now in the process of finding out where the other infection is. It could be in my gums, my bowels, or some other place. I'm starting with my teeth and gums.

I thought the infection might be in my mouth. Therefore, I went to a dentist who could x-ray my mouth and tell me if I had any cavities in my gums that might indicate infection. He has an x-ray unit that travels around your jaw and provides you with a single x-ray of all your teeth and gums in a panorama presentation. He found no sign of infection. However, he found one remaining filling that might have mercury in it. I thought they were all gone. Since this was a tooth that had a previous root canal procedure that I had not done anything about, I decided to just have the tooth pulled. Coincidentally, my latest hair analysis showed a slight increase in mercury. My last previous hair analysis indicated a big drop in mercury and only a slight trace. I am now scheduled for another DMPS chelation treatment and I'll have my urine checked also.

Recognizing and avoiding toxins in your environment is the most difficult problem I have had in my recovery period. I've been doing this now for over seven years and you'd think that I would have it figured out by now. Alas, such is not the case. Let me tell you of my recent experience so you may understand the scope of the problem.

I have had three setbacks in the last two or three months. Each time I can trace it to a toxin. Now you might wonder how I can do that. Well, because I eat the same foods everyday and my environment rarely changes. So all I have to do is look for the one item that changed.

Recently, we brought our Ms Pac-man video game out of storage and put it on our rear deck. I would play the game for a couple of hours at a time. Now, I'm barefoot and the only thing I wear is shorts because the weather here is very warm. Then, I had a setback. At first I could not figure it out. But after another day I felt some lumps on the bottom of my left foot. I had Glenna look at them and they were three little blisters. I had seen a small black widow spider in a web from the Pac-man to the floor but I ignored it. However, I think he bit me. That's the only explanation I have for the setback and the blisters on my foot.

Another time, Glenna sprayed the roses which are located adjacent to our rear deck. Naturally I was inside all the time she was spraying. However, I wanted to play Pac-man so I went out later in the day and played for a couple of hours. Within a few more hours, I had a setback. Now you wouldn't think that the spray from the roses several hours earlier could hurt me. However, I'm convinced it did.

The third item occurred when we ate out. We ate dinner out at a restaurant I have been to before and they have told me that they do not use MSG. However, a restaurant may use ingredients that contain MSG that they are not aware of. At any rate, that meal caused me to have a setback.

Oh yes, I almost forgot. There was a fourth one. This one might really surprise you. I don't eat cheese very often and then I don't eat much, so I never had a problem before from eating cheese. I bought some goat cheese because I thought that would be better for me. I ate a bunch of it and I had a setback. I couldn't believe the cheese was the problem. So a few days later, I did it again and I had another setback. I read the label again that shows the ingredients. Included was the word "enzymes." Sometimes the word "enzymes" is another word for MSG. You never really know. In this case, it was.

Again, I tell you this because avoiding toxins is your most difficult problem. I wonder where I would be now if I had not had the many setbacks that I have had over the last few years. The moral of the story is that I should follow my own advice better and avoid anything that is even questionable. At any rate, I just wanted to share these recent experiences so you might have a glimpse of the problem.

Update – May 2004 on Water Filters

I am not an expert on water filters but I think very highly of Dr. David Williams and his *"Alternatives"* newsletter. He recommends a Waterwise 9000 Distiller for drinking water. It is expensive – around $400, but it may be worth it. You can call Toll-Free 1-800-888-1415 or go online at:

drdavidwilliamscatalog.com

CHAPTER 8

DETOXIFY THE BODY

Part Two of My Program

You cannot, in my opinion, improve your ALS condition without doing many things. However, if there is one thing that's more important than the others, it is detoxifying the body. If you have a medically untreatable illness, like ALS or something similar, my theory is that you no doubt have an accumulation of toxins in your body.

Unless the toxins are removed, you have little or no hope of restoring your health.

There may be a thousand ways to detox the body. "Eric, I've told you ten million times not to exaggerate." Well, maybe that is an exaggeration, but there are many, many ways. I am not an expert in this field and I don't claim to know all the ways this can be done. I will tell you of the ones I know about, most of which I have experienced.

Detox can be accomplished by diet, drinking plenty of pure water, bathing in naturally hot mineral water, body massage, chelation therapy, fasting, colonic irrigation or colon hydrotherapy, steam baths, and now a new one to me bathing in Bentonite clay to name a few of the more common ones.

To start with, I would recommend a comprehensive blood test and a hair analysis to find out what your primary toxins are. If you have ALS or some other neurological condition and a mouthful of amalgams, then you most certainly have some mercury in your system. If you have a significant amount of mercury, chelation should be strongly considered.

Chelation Therapy

What is it? Chelate means to bind with or combine with another element such as metal. Chelation therapy that I'm talking about is a treatment where a substance called Di Mercapto Propane Sulphonate (DMPS) is put into your blood stream by injection that takes about ten or fifteen minutes. The DMPS chelates or binds with the mercury and both are filtered out of your system. Normally, this involves 10 or 20 treatments. Customarily they check your urine for mercury content after several treatments. The urine is accumulated for several hours following a treatment and then sent to the lab. Mercury may not show up in a normal urinalysis, that is, without prior chelation therapy. However, if you have any mercury at all in your system, I assure you it will show up in your urine immediately after chelation.

Please note that chelation therapy is normally associated with improving your circulation. However, they use a different chelating agent called EDTA for that purpose.

EDTA was originally created to remove **lead** from the many shipyard workers who developed lead poisoning during World War II in the late 1940's.

DMPS was created a decade or more later to remove **mercury**.

Chelation therapy with either EDTA or DMPS is approved by the FDA but not by the AMA. Therefore, chelation is not practiced by mainstream medical doctors. The reason for this is simple economics. Chelation is an inexpensive substitute for all the expensive procedures like angioplasties and open heart bypass surgery, etc. According to a recent Danish study, 58 out of 65 heart patients who received chelation therapy while they were on the waiting list for bypass surgery did not need the bypass after several months of chelation.

If you are interested in more details on chelation therapy, then I would recommend you read a book that I have recently discovered: *"Forty Something Forever, A Consumer's Guide to Chelation Therapy and other Heart-Savers"* by Harold and Arline Brecher. This book not only contains a great deal of information on chelation, but also a lot of other general health information. It's a great book.

Anyone interested in finding a physician trained in chelation therapy can call ACAM.

The American College for Advancement in Medicine (ACAM) is a not-for-profit medical society dedicated to educating physicians and other healthcare professionals on the latest findings and emerging procedures in preventive/nutritional medicine. These doctors also do chelation treatments. ACAM represents more than 1,000 physicians in many countries. My Dr. Rouzier is an ACAM doctor. He is exactly what I want in a doctor. He is a medical doctor specializing in prevention and alternative treatments. To find one in your area, you can contact them at the address below or look on their website:

> American College for Advancement in Medicine
> 23121 Verdugo Dr., Suite 204
> Laguna Hills, California 92653
> Phone (949) 583-7666 or
> Toll Free Outside CA: (800) 532-3688

> Here is their website: *www.acam.org*

Restoring Bacteria in the Colon

This isn't exactly detox, but essential to your detox program.

I ordered a book and videotape from a neurologist in Florida who claimed success in treating MS patients by improving the "integrity of the gut." Those are his words. What he means is, restoring the digestion system, including the colon, to a healthy condition. You see, in order to get the ultimate benefit from the food you eat and the supplements you take, the digestive system must be in good working condition. Additionally, your digestive system must be in good working order in order to maximize any detox treatment. I believe that this doctor has the right idea. His videotape was very convincing. It just stands to reason that your digestive system must be in good working order. One of the common problems with our digestive system is brought on by the heavy use of prescription drugs such as antibiotics. There are good bacteria and bad bacteria in our systems. When you take an antibiotic drug, it destroys *all* bacteria, both good and bad. It is essential for your digestive system to have good bacteria. Unfortunately, antibiotic drugs can't tell good bacteria from bad bacteria. After taking an antibiotic drug, you should restore the good bacteria in your system. I know this is another shot at the medical doctors, but they deserve it. Have you ever had a medical doctor tell you anything about restoring good bacteria to your colon? If you have, yours is a rare experience. I never have. One way to restore bacteria is by taking a product called Ultra Flora Plus DF by Metagenics. The label goes on to say "Dairy-Free NCFM Strain Advanced Probiotic Nutrition & Probio-Saccharide Factor (FOS) – Guaranteed 2.25 billion Lactobacillus acidophilus and 2.25 billion Bifidobacterium infantis per serving at expiration."

Recently, I have had trouble with loose bowels again. Coincidentally, I started drinking buttermilk again. I had not had any buttermilk since I started my program in 1996. Buttermilk has some of the same ingredients that Ultra Flora Plus DF has. In other words, it too will help restore good bacteria to your colon. It is hard for me to drink a lot of water and therefore I forget to take my Ultra Flora. However, I love buttermilk. I wasn't doing this on purpose because I really had no idea what the effect would be. However, after drinking buttermilk for a couple of weeks, my loose bowel problem was completely eliminated. I have now gone over five months without a BM accident and that, says Glenna, is great news!! Remember that Glenna is in charge of the clean up committee.

Note: Ultra Flora should be taken in between meals such as an hour before or two hours after a meal. I recently found a good time to take it. When I first get up in the morning, Glenna brings me a glass of Ultra Flora to drink at that time. It is usually an hour before I eat breakfast, so that's a good time and I don't forget to do it.

Note: Another really good probiotic is Intestinal Care DF by Ethical Nutrients, also a division of Metagenics.

Note: The above discussion about the colon is good basic information. However, I have learned a lot more recently about our digestive system and it is in the March 2004 Update at the end of this chapter.

Colon Hydrotherapy

Your colon is just like the plumbing from your kitchen sink. Over the years, grease, etc. can build up on the walls of your plumbing and eventually stop it up completely. What do you do when that happens? You call in the Roto-Rooter man to clean it out. Colon hydrotherapy is the same general idea. Just like in your plumbing, you can have a partial blockage in your colon. This can occur in a pocket or a bend in your colon. You probably would never be aware of it. However, this can create a source of toxins and threaten your health. I have read that therapists have removed as much as several pounds of material that had been stuck in the colon for a long time. I know that sounds hard to believe, but I'm sure it is true.

Some people think it is a good idea to have colon hydrotherapy done periodically even if you're healthy; seems reasonable to me. I know, you thought that once "that stuff" got in your bladder and colon, it would be eliminated from your body. Well, that's not so.

Have you ever picked up a tortoise in the desert and had it urinate on you? They do this as a defense hoping you will put them down and most people do immediately. Those in the know will tell you *not* to pick them up for that reason. When they urinate, they lose all that fluid. By not urinating, they hold that fluid in their system and it is recycled. The tortoise knows that water in the desert is a treasure.

I know the recycling works this way from my own experience. Normally, I'm like anyone else, after a couple of beers I have to urinate. However, one time we were dove hunting in the desert near Calexico in 120-degree weather. After the hunt, my friends and I sat down in the shade of a tree to guzzle a few beers. I realized the next day when thinking back that I never urinated that afternoon until about 8 PM. Prior to that, I'm certain I had at least six beers and probably more like eight or nine. Normally I would have urinated several times after drinking that much beer. However, I did not go for several hours. Well, where did the liquid go? It was recycled. The body automatically does this in that kind of heat. The camel does the same thing only he is better at it.

Unfortunately, when the fluid is drawn out of your bladder and colon and recycled back into your system, it carries many toxins with it. Therefore, in order to eliminate toxins, we need a free-flowing system and plenty of water to avoid recycling.

Colon hydrotherapy was one of the first things I did when I started my program. At first, I had this done three times a week for about a month, twice a week for a month and then once a week for about three or four months. I still continue to have this done once every month or two.

When I first started these treatments, they made me feel good. I can't tell you how exactly, only that I had a gut feeling that they were helping me. As it turns out, they must have been, because that's when I started improving.

The liver filters toxins and other debris from your blood stream. It acts just like the filter in your swimming pool. Your liver, just like your pool filter, can get plugged up with debris. This can cause havoc with your health. You need to help your liver cleanse itself particularly when you're going through any detox program. To accomplish this, my colon therapist had me take one ounce of pure fresh lemon juice with one ounce of 100% virgin olive oil. Put the lemon juice and olive oil in a blender with a couple of ice cubes and blend. This is a noxious drink or a lousy margarita. To make it a little more palatable, add two or three drops of the sugar substitute I previously recommended (Stevia Extract). You take this drink before bedtime the night before a colon treatment. Sleep on your right side all night. This helps your liver detox.

Bowel Movements

In addition to colonic hydrotherapy treatments, I think it is critical to have frequent bowel movements. All else that you're doing may not be effective without proper elimination. The toxins from your system can best be eliminated from the body with frequent bowel movements. I have always gone once a day and occasionally twice a day. I continue to do that now even though I have to use an enema frequently. My latest innovation in the department of BMs involves Metamucil. I have found that taking Metamucil twice a day helps me prevent accidents by having a BM twice a day. I take Metamucil once in the morning before my breakfast and again in the evening before dinner. This works great.

Update – March 2004

There is a really great substitute for Metamucil that I recently learned about. **It is psyllium,** and it is available at most health food stores. It's a lot cheaper than Metamucil. Psyllium is the main ingredient in Metamucil but without the sugar and food coloring that is completely unnecessary. I now take psyllium twice a day and I prefer it.

Note: While we are on the subject of BMs, let me make a suggestion that might help you. I use a raised potty-chair over the toilet. I found it to be very awkward to sit on until I lowered the front legs about two inches. This creates a slight angle forward for the toilet seat. I find that to be much more comfortable to get up and down from.

Hot Mineral Water Baths

Whether or not bathing in hot mineral water is beneficial to your health is controversial. Of course, everything I'm doing is controversial. However, I'm sure you will really question this procedure. With that in mind, let me tell you another family story. "No, no, not *another* one?" Yes, yes, because this is the only thing I know of that might prove the value of mineral water bathing.

I know you're wondering if all these stories can be true. You will really be wondering after this next one. Let me assure you that I am not artistically inclined, have almost zero imagination and I was taught by my mother to always tell the truth. What I am saying is that I simply don't have the imagination to dream these up. I say this ahead of time because this story is hard to believe.

In the mid 1950's my mother and stepfather, George Ritchie, bought 40 acres near Mammoth Lakes, California called Casa Diablo Hot Springs. Included on the land were a house, a two-car garage, gasoline service station, and a restaurant-bar building. In addition to the buildings, there was a natural mineral hot springs on the property, hence the name Casa Diablo Hot Springs. My folks made this their home. George ran the gas station and garage repair and my mother handled the bar and restaurant. This is cold country and it snows a lot (7000 feet elevation). George improvised a system to heat the house. He ran a pipe from a steam vent near the hot springs over to the house. Then, into the house and into two 50 gallon metal drums that were located in the back room. This provided ample heat for the home in the coldest of weather. For his next trick, he ran a pipe from the hot spring water into the house and connected it to the bathtub. Alas, a natural hot mineral water bathing tub right in the house. My step-dad was pretty clever even if I do say so myself.

About this same time, my Uncle Harvey (my mother's brother) developed a really bad skin problem. Something I've never seen before or since. His skin turned a dark purple color like a beet all over his body. His skin was like leather and would crack and bleed. He went from skin doctor to skin doctor to no avail. Harvey lived in North Hollywood, California about 300 miles to the south. Harvey came up to Casa Diablo to visit my mother. George suggested to Harvey that he stay there a while and bathe in the tub with the hot mineral water. Well, nothing else was working, not even Harvey, so he decided to stay and try it. After about a month, Harvey's skin began to improve. Naturally, that encouraged him to continue soaking in the mineral water. Harvey would soak in the water about one hour every evening before bedtime. One night Harvey was in bathing and George and my mother were in the other room. Suddenly Harvey shouted out "George, George, come quick." Harvey was in the tub and blood was pouring out of his left leg from a cavity the size of an egg. At first the blood was dark red, almost black, and then it changed to a normal red. A black ball of tissue was lying in the tub that had come out of Harvey's leg leaving the cavity. From that day on Harvey's improvement was more rapid and in a few more weeks he returned to normal.

Now those are the facts. I saw Harvey both before and after this happened. I know nothing else had anything to do with his recovery. We can only speculate on what caused this. However, I'm certain that whatever was in that ball was toxic. It could have been a spider bite or something similar, but nonetheless, some form of toxin. Maybe the whole damn bug was in there, who knows?

"Well, Eric, that is quite a story, but what is the conclusion?" The conclusion is that hot mineral water bathing can eliminate toxins from the body.

If you recall your history, the Spanish explorer, Ponce de Leon, was searching for the "Fountain of Youth" and never found it. He never found it, because he didn't know what he was looking for.

Is a hot springs a fountain? I would say so in the broad sense of the word. Sometimes there are geysers in hot springs. A geyser would certainly qualify for a fountain. Does bathing in mineral hot springs restore your youth? No, not exactly. They can't turn back the calendar. However, as in Harvey's case, they can extend your life. The hot springs at Casa Diablo unquestionably added 15 years to Harvey's life. Could it be said then that hot springs are the true "Fountain of Youth?" I believe that could be true!

I want to point out that the water used to treat Harvey was pure unpolluted, unchlorinated hot springs water. You may not be able to find that. All public swimming and bathing pools must be chlorinated to the best of my knowledge. Whether or not you would have the same success bathing in chlorinated hot springs water is unknown to me.

Diet and Supplements

The body will tend to detoxify itself automatically but at a very slow rate. The rate of detox can be accelerated by certain foods and certain supplements. I have read about cilantro. It is a green leafy plant similar to parsley. It can bind with mercury and carry the mercury out of your system. I believe that the antioxidants A, E and C will also have some effect on removal of mercury. If you have had a hair analysis and you have a low amount of mercury, as I did, then you might elect to go this route instead of chelation therapy. If you have a lot of mercury in your system, then chelation is the only way to go.

I started my program in January of 1997. I did not know then what I know now about ALS. I did not have a hair analysis then. I didn't know about amalgams. I finally had my amalgams removed in March 1998. Then I learned about hair analysis. I had my first hair analysis in May 1998. On their scale of low, medium, and high, I was between low and medium for mercury toxicity. For that reason, I did not do chelation, but continued my program of supplements and added cilantro for a while. Approximately a year later, in July of 1999, I had another hair analysis. It indicated my mercury was at the low end of the spectrum. It had gone from 1.12 to .14. Additionally, my lead went from .79 to .35. Arsenic went from .068 to .031. This was a happy day for me. I knew what I was doing was working for certain. The hair analysis report also told me that my manganese, chromium, iodine, lithium, and sulfur were all too low so I immediately added those to my supplements.

According to a recent article I read, alpha-lipoic acid is effective in binding with and removing mercury. They tout it as the Cadillac of all antioxidants.

Water

It is absolutely necessary to drink a certain amount of water to keep your body from dehydrating, to maintain your digestive system, and to flush toxins from your system. Even the medical doctors agree on this one. It is universally accepted that we should drink a lot of water. The usual amount recommended is eight glasses a day. Now I'm not going to tell you that I do this. This is one where I fail miserably. I have a devil of a time drinking water. To drink eight glasses of water in one day is beyond my capacity. I have never done that in my whole life except on a few unusual days where I was working in the sun on a hot day.

This is another example of how we are all different. My system simply does not require a lot of water. I have been on all day hiking sojourns without ever drinking a drop. However, I always carry food to eat that contains fluid, such as a fresh orange or an apple. At any rate, I do believe you should drink as much water as possible. If you can handle eight glasses a day, then I recommend you do it. Make sure its pure water. Distilled water stored in a glass container is best.

Body Massage

Yes, even body massage has its place here, as it will help you detox. Anything that increases your circulation, particularly your circulation down deep in the muscles, can help you detox. A body massage, especially a deep body massage, affects your circulation. I did this once or twice a week for a couple of months early in my program. I still have one occasionally.

Fasting

This is still another way to detoxify the body of various poisons. It may not be suitable for people with ALS because they may have already suffered weight loss and muscle atrophy. However, I want to mention it to you as one possibility. Paul Bragge, a health enthusiast from many years ago, recommended fasting for 36 hours once a week. You do this by simply avoiding your normal meals for one day. In other words, if you had your last meal at 8 PM on Monday and your next meal at 8 AM Wednesday, you would have fasted for 36 hours. During that time, you would drink only liquids; you want to drink a lot of liquids. Some people drink only water and others drink only fresh raw vegetable juice from a juicer. Either way, you're allowing your body to rest from all the normal work of digesting. This allows your body to concentrate on detoxification.

You might question whether or not this is effective. All I can offer for proof is that Paul Bragge died at age 95. Therefore, he must have been doing something right. Of even greater interest is the fact that he was surfing in Hawaii at age 95 when he was killed in a surfing accident. If you had to die, what better way is there? That's even better than being shot to death at age 95 by a jealous husband!

Breathing

The veins carry the blood back to the lungs and the blood contains impurities. The lungs remove some of the impurities and they are exhaled. You inhale fresh air containing oxygen and that refreshes the blood.

Then, the refreshed blood is carried throughout your system of arteries, muscles and organs. This entire process is only as effective as your breathing. Therefore, it may be a good idea to perform a deep breathing exercise several times a day.

Update – Eliminating another toxin – March 2004

Previously I have discussed the fact that my improvement over the last several years has been very slow. At this point in my progress I really believe that I should have been improving at a faster rate. It has long been my suspicion that there is another toxin in my body that I don't know about. Now, at long last, I think I have discovered what it is.

There are several things that can get into our digestive tract that are either toxic themselves, or they create toxins.

1. Mildew can create toxic vapors that you breathe.
2. Fungus can be on some foods that you eat such as grain, potatoes, pasta, flour and yeast.
3. Bad bacteria. All of us have both good and bad bacteria in our digestive tract. Most of us, including me, have too much of the bad bacteria because of antibiotics.
4. Mycotoxins. These little bugs get in your intestines from food that you eat. I have read that 85% of all PALS have Mycotoxins in their system.

Doug Kaufmann has written a book called *"The Germ that Causes Cancer."* Remember now, cancer is caused by toxins also. I recommend that if you have ALS or any other neurological illness, you should read this book. Also, anyone with Irritable Bowel Syndrome or Irritable Bowel Disease should read it.

There's another book called *"Patient Heal Thyself"* by Jordan S. Rubin, N.M.D, C.N.C. He has the same theory as Kaufmann.

A third source of information on this same subject can be found on Linda Paulhus' new website. She has just created about a twenty page website just for PALS. She has accumulated much more information about ALS.

This is a must-view website:

http://www.alsalternative.com/

Linda has also told me about a lady doctor in Boston, Dr. Menqi Xiu, who is successfully treating ALS patients with a two-step system:

1. Detox the liver, kidneys, and the colon.
2. Restore the body with Lutimax.

All of the above people believe generally the same thing. That is, most of us have toxic bugs in our gut and they **must be eliminated.**

There are many, many ways to eliminate the parasites and their toxic effect from your intestines. Kaufmann suggests a diet for two to four weeks of no grain of any kind among other things and an antibiotic for two to four weeks. The diet is basically a no starch, no sugar diet. Then, follow that with several **natural antibiotics.** Take one natural antibiotic for thirty days and then change to another one. Some of those recommended are:

1. Colloidal Silver
2. Oil of Oregano
3. Natural Raw Garlic
4. Olive Leaf Extract (The best is by Seagate.)

The real beauty of these natural antibiotics is that they kill only the bad fungus and bad bacteria, but they don't kill the good bacteria. To the best of my knowledge, the pharmaceutical antibiotics kill **all** the bacteria including the good bacteria.

Update – New Treatments – March 2004

Another PALS called me from New Jersey and told me that he was once unable to talk but after many treatments with a Phoenix, Arizona doctor he could now talk again. I called the Phoenix doctor and learned about the two treatments that he was doing. They referred me to the manufacturer of the equipment that is used. I called the manufacturer and they gave me the name of a doctor in my area who had purchased the two items of equipment. The two treatments are Bionic Cleansing and a Laser Treatment.

The manufacturer of the two instruments is Erchonia Medical, Inc. For more information, call Energy Balance Resources at 4270 Mt. Davis Avenue, San Diego, California 92117. Phone 1-866-522-5262. Web address is:

www.4ebr.com

They will provide you with the name of a doctor trained to use this equipment.

Bionic Cleansing

This is a Phase One treatment that will detoxify your body. It may sound crazy, but it works. You put your feet in a tub of water with an electrical instrument and it draws toxins out of your body through your feet. You know it is working because after a few minutes the water will change color in accordance with the type of toxin being eliminated.

Laser Treatment

This is also very mysterious, but again it works. This is simply a laser beam that the doctor will shine on your body and move around. I would call it a stimulator. It will stimulate your nerves, your muscles, your brain and your body organs. For that reason, it is a little bit of Phase One and Phase Two. When it stimulates your organs, it may be helping your body to eliminate toxins. My doctor does arm muscle testing to evaluate the effect of the laser treatment. Now I know first hand by the muscle testing that this one works also.

Human Growth Hormone

I have now been taking a daily shot of HGH for a long time. It is a little expensive, but I know it works for me. It comes in many forms but I selected a throwaway syringe. It has no preservatives because you mix it in the syringe just before you apply it. The needle is so fine that most of the time I don't even feel it. My wife, who would never give me a regular shot of anything, gives me this shot everyday with no problem. You can only obtain this with a prescription from your MD.

Starbucks

Now you're going to laugh when I tell you this one. However, I am dead serious. I truly believe that the drink that I buy at Starbucks everyday is helping me. They make a chai tea latte with soy milk. Chai tea is a black tea which contains antioxidants. Additionally, Starbucks adds many spices such as ginger, cinnamon, etc. Now I have no idea whether it is the tea, the spices, or the soy milk, but I don't care. Strangely, two or three hours after a latte I feel a lot stronger. Additionally, when I check my pH at the same time it is higher. You can draw your own conclusion but I am still drinking my Chai tea latte everyday.

Starbucks and Trader Joe's sell a mix for chai tea latte that you can make at home with your own soy milk.

Bentonite Clay & LL's Magnetic Clay

LL's Magnetic Clay may be the best Bentonite Clay for bathing and detoxifying the body.

A group of people caring for autistic children applied this new treatment with some success. Apparently autism is caused by toxins just like toxins cause ALS and many other neurological illnesses.

Here is a website for more information:

http://www.evenbetternow.com/autism.html

When you reach the website, scroll down to "#7 Detoxify heavy metals" and then read from there on for several pages. The real "meat" of the article is under the heading "LL's Magnetic Clay."

More information on LL's Magnetic Clay may be found on the following website:

http://www.evenbetternow.com/

For more information about ALS and LL's Magnetic Clay, go to the following website:

http://www.evenbetternow.com/als.html
If you just want to order the clay,
you can call toll free (877) 562-6039.

I called the phone number for LL's and talked with Andrea Nichol. She was most helpful and informative. I told her I did not have a bathtub; only a shower. She told me I could do a foot bath with one-half cup of clay powder and that would be about 70% as effective as a full bath.

I did one foot bath for twelve minutes. My feet were very tingly for a long time after the bath and I just felt very good. I cannot describe exactly how or why.

I did my second foot bath for fifteen minutes. A short time after the foot bath, I realized I could move my toes. So what's remarkable about that Eric? Well, I have not been able to move my toes for the last several years. I didn't really realize that until I was able to move them again.

I have never had an experience like this immediately following any other detox treatment. Therefore, I want to recommend that you consider the clay bath or clay foot bath. I cannot recommend anything for any one of you, but if I were you, I would sure look into it more and consult your healthcare professional.

Based on my experience and what I've read, **THE CLAY MAY BE A BETTER DETOX TREATMENT THAN CHELATION OR BIONIC CLEANSING OR MAYBE ANY OTHER TREATMENT.** It certainly is inexpensive and simple.

Detox Warning!

I am not recommending any of these treatments for any individual. You should work with a healthcare professional. Even so, I want to remind you that anytime you do any detox treatment, you may get worse before you get better. In order to minimize the bad effect of a detox treatment, it is suggested that you have a nutritious diet plus supplements before, during and after any detox treatments.

I received a very sad e-mail recently from a PALS' caregiver spouse. He told me his wife had just died. Now that's sad enough, but here is the real heartbreaker. He told me that she had been on a "heavy detox" treatment under the care of a medical doctor and she was actually improving just before she died.

Obviously you must be very careful when undergoing any detox treatment. However, if you have ALS or something similar, you will die if you don't detox. I would rather go down fighting than go down like a wimp.

Most detox treatments, other than colonic hydrotherapy, create an additional burden as your body eliminates the toxins. Depending on how much mercury is in your system and/or how far along your ALS condition has progressed, all detox treatments should not be done too hastily. The toxins must be removed if you are going to live, but too much too soon could cause serious problems.

Here's one way that will give you a clue as to how your body is functioning in eliminating toxins. Measure the pH of your urine. If your body is working properly, it should be eliminating acids and the pH of your urine should be below 7.0; it should be around 5.8. As your body detoxifies, there should be, eventually, less acid in your urine and the pH level should go up to around 7.0. At the same time, the pH of your saliva should be improving also.

CHAPTER 9

DIET & DIETARY SUPPLEMENTS

Part Three of My Program

Establishing a proper diet is critical to the success of any program to improve your health. Some people may question that statement. However, it is hard for me to understand. Tell me this, what is wrong with the idea that good nutrition can heal the body? After all, you are what you eat, drink, think, say and do. Everyone knows that the absence of certain foods and minerals can cause serious health problems. Conversely, it should stand to reason that the eating of high-quality and nutritious food would lead to excellent health. Therefore, it is my firm belief that a good diet is paramount to good health and healing.

We have already discussed proper diet in Part One. That same diet will provide proper nourishment *and* avoid many toxins. All we need to talk about now is supplements. Supplements include vitamins. Vitamins are the heart of the nutrition in the food we eat.

Before we review my list of supplements, let's talk about why anyone should take supplements. According to a government study, not one person in the research received 100% of RDA's (recommended daily allowance) of all vitamins and minerals in their normal daily diet. RDA's are not the *optimum* amount but rather the *minimum* amount recommended. There are many reasons for this; everything has changed from a hundred years ago in the food you buy at the market. The food is grown in soil with depleted minerals, pesticides are used, the food is harvested prematurely, processing of foods, etc. The only way to be sure you're getting sufficient amounts of vitamins and minerals is to take supplements, or grow everything yourself. Additionally, many studies have shown the benefit of taking larger doses of vitamins for better health.

Another powerful reason for taking vitamins and supplements is that many of them are what we call antioxidants. Antioxidants are the enemy of free radicals. What are free radicals? You will find these free radicals down at the level of atoms and molecules. Free radicals are like 'loose canons' in your system traveling throughout your body attacking healthy cells. You might also wonder where they come from. They are created by toxins such as chemicals, heavy metals, tobacco smoke, and many more. It is well established that free radicals in your system can cause many health problems. In fact, studies have shown that there is a deficiency of an antioxidant enzyme in ALS patients. That enzyme is superoxide dismutase (SOD). Therefore, there is an unquestionable need for antioxidants in the ALS patient. Remember, free radicals are the problem and antioxidants limit the life span of free radicals. Therefore, a vitamin and mineral supplement program including many antioxidants is essential for good health today.

Here is a list of what I have been taking. It has been modified slightly from when I started in January of 1997. I do not suggest that anyone follow this regimen without the supervision of a MD or some other healthcare professional. The supplements you take should be customized to your precise needs. Additionally, your tolerance for all of these may be different from mine. I have had to make several changes due to my intolerance for some supplements:

Vitamin A – 24000 iu
Vitamin B-1 – 200 mg
Vitamin B-12 – 2000 mcg
Vitamin D – 400 iu
Vitamin E – 3600 iu
B Complex with Vitamin B-1 – 50 mg

Calcium – Two Tablets of Cal Apatite 1000 (By Metagenics)

DHEA – 300 mg

Flax Seed Oil – 14 g

Ginkgo Biloba Extract – 120 mg

Glucosamine & Chondroitin

Glucosamine – 1000 mg

Chondroitin – 800 mg

Grape Seed Extract – 200 mg (Similar to Pycnogenol)

Alpha-lipoic acid – 300 mg

NADH – 5 mg

Coenzyme Q-10 – 60 mg

Selenium – 200 mcg

Ultra Potent Vitamin C – 2000 mg (By Metagenics)

Multigenics Powder – 10 g (By Metagenics – Multi Vitamins & Multi Minerals)

Ultra Clear Sustain – 60 g (By Metagenics – Sustained Nutrition Beverage Mix – Gastrointestinal Support Program)

Phyto Complete – Synergistic Phytonutrient Complex – One Scoop (By Metagenics)

Colloidal Minerals – One Tablespoon

Chromium Picolinate – 800mcg

The above last three items, Phyto Complete, Colloidal Minerals and Chromium Picolinate, have just been added as a direct result of my latest hair analysis. There are so many good supplements that you probably can't take them all. However, if I were starting over, I would consider adding PABA (para amino benzoic acid), L-Carnitine, Glutathione, and Phosphatidylserine. These are said to have great restorative powers on the nervous system. These are contained in my IV treatment that I'm currently taking.

I don't like to take any supplement without knowing the reason for taking it. You should not take any of the above supplements without knowing why you're taking them. As I have said before, you should work with a nutritionist. Let me tell you why I take these supplements.

Multi-Vitamins and Minerals plus B-Complex and B-1

All my life I have probably eaten more fresh vegetables and fresh fruit than the average person. In spite of that, I think we need a multi-vitamin and mineral supplement just for general well being.

I began wearing glasses for close work at my desk when I was about 35 years old. I found I could not read without them. At age 47, I was still wearing glasses. I had been taking a multi-vitamin for several years. Something I read caused me to add B-Complex with 100 units of B-1. I was afraid I might be duplicating some of the multi-vitamin, but I did it anyway.

Two or three months later, I was reading at my desk and realized that I was having a problem reading. I took my glasses off and tried reading. I found I could read better without them. Well, guess what! I quit wearing them. I'm now 71 years old and I've never put them back on until recently. According to my optometrist, I have 20/20 vision. Given the proper lighting, I can read the stock market quotes in the daily newspaper without glasses. However, I don't always have proper lighting, so I use my reading glasses for that one purpose only.

That's why, to this day, I take a multi-vitamin and the B Complex, but with one modification. I found that the B-100 Complex would sometimes increase my anxiety level. I would get very nervous and jittery. Therefore, I changed to a B-50 Complex. This seems to work quite well for me.

Vitamin B-1

My alternative treatment doctor recommended 300 B-1 daily. B-1 is supposed to be good for your nervous system. I have found that I can take 200 B-1 in addition to one tablet of 50 B-Complex and not have an anxiety problem.

Vitamin A, E, C Pycnogenol or Grape Seed Extract & Q-10

I've read that most health problems are the result of free radicals in your system. All of the above are antioxidants and the enemy of free radicals.

If I could take only one or two vitamins in this group, it would be E and Pycnogenol. I don't mean to brag, but at 71 years old, I do not need

Viagra. I have taken Vitamin E off and on for around 30 years. When I take Vitamin E, there is an increase in this department. When I do not take Vitamin E, then there is a definite lack of adequate function in this same department. Vitamin E has unquestionably improved my sexual performance. I figure if you can tell the difference a vitamin makes in just one part of your body, then it must be good for you overall as well.

I have read that Pycnogenol may be as much as fifty times more potent than Vitamin E and may be the only antioxidant capable of penetrating the blood/brain barrier.

Vitamin B-12 & D

We seem to need more of these two vitamins as we get older.

Calcium

ALS patients seem to have a shortage of Calcium. Therefore, there is an obvious need for this supplement.

DHEA

DHEA is not a vitamin or mineral supplement. It is a hormone normally produced by your body. When you are young, your body produces adequate amounts of DHEA. Apparently, as a part of the aging process, your body produces less and less as you get older. Studies have shown a direct relationship between reduced levels of DHEA and many diseases of old age such as arthritis, etc. The theory, based on these studies, is that if you maintain your DHEA at a level equal to that of a young person, you might avoid many old age problems and even live longer.

You can buy DHEA at the health food store but the maximum dose in one tablet is 50. Well, if you really have a low level of DHEA like I did, then 50 is a drop in the bucket. The normal level of DHEA in a young man is somewhere around 400 to 600. My blood test indicated mine was 50. You can see why I take 300 units a day. You can also see the need to have a blood test to determine what your supplement should be.

I've been taking DHEA for about five years now. There's no way to know, but I attribute Vitamin E and DHEA to my not needing Viagra.

I think 300 is a little low for me and I'll be going to a new doctor soon to discuss increasing my DHEA to around 600 units a day. In order to get optimum results, I think I need that much and I wish now that I had been taking more all along.

One last comment about DHEA; you can buy it at the vitamin store or from the pharmacy. I think the pharmacy grade of DHEA may be of higher quality plus you can get a higher dosage in a single capsule.

Flax Seed Oil

This is a source of Omega-3 fatty acids: essential for good health.

Ginkgo Biloba Extract

I can't remember why I take this one, Glenna, do you know? Glenna replies, "It's for your memory stupid!" Oh yeh – just kidding.

I don't take this for ALS. This is supposed to be good for the brain and more specifically for your memory. I believe it works and that my memory has actually improved in the last four or five years. To give you an example, I was thinking recently about my grandmother and could not remember her last husband's name. He was number four. She outlived four husbands. Anyway, I couldn't remember his name because I hadn't thought about it for 40 years. Then, I said to myself, "I'll think about it later." Remember how I told you that works? Well, about four or five days later his name came to me out of the blue. His name was Ed Welton. So you see, I believe my memory is probably better than a few years ago.

Glucosamine & Chondroitin

These are not for ALS either. These two supplements are supposed to be good for arthritis. I have had severe arthritis in my left shoulder for many years. My arthritis has been improving ever since the removal of my amalgams *and* since I began taking these two supplements.

Alpha-lipoic acid (ALA)

I have been taking 50 or 100 units of ALA since around 1995. However, I just raised it to 300 units after reading a very interesting article on it. The article said that ALA was the ultimate antioxidant and that it worked synergistically with other antioxidants such as E and C. ALA can also chelate excess metals.

ALA is another substance that not only occurs in some foods, but the body also produces it. And again, it is a substance that the body produces less of as you get older.

ALA deficiency has been linked to muscle atrophy and brain atrophy.

ALA is a tremendous antioxidant and a protector of the nervous system. Also, it may help regenerate nerves.

NADH

This has something to do with regeneration of nerve and brain cells.

Selenium

ALS patients seem to have a shortage of Selenium. Therefore, there is an obvious need for this supplement.

Multigenics Powder

This is simply my multi-vitamin and mineral supplement.

Ultra Clear Sustain

I took this for the first year or so to re-establish the integrity of the gut. This is also a source of protein. I'm not currently taking this.

Raw Vegetable Juice

I previously mentioned that I add all these supplements to a veggie drink. I've told you why I take all the supplements, and I think I should tell you why I take the vegetable juice also. One of the primary universal rules of nature is "Stay as close to Mother Nature as possible." This applies to all phases of your life but most importantly to your diet. In the beginning, centuries ago, we undoubtedly ate fruit that we picked right off of the tree and vegetables that we harvested directly from the field. They would be fresh, uncontaminated, and raw. When you alter them in any way, even cooking, you have moved away from nature. When you eat a raw vegetable, you are eating a living plant. When you eat a cooked vegetable, you are eating a dead plant. Some health benefit is no doubt lost in the cooking process. Well, fine, let's eat a lot of raw veggies. Whoa – hold on 'pardner,' raw veggies don't taste good and it takes a long time to chew them up. What can we do about that? Well, we can buy a vegetable juicer and make juice from the veggies and drink that. That is not exactly nature's way, but pretty damn close to it. Vitamins and supplements obviously have their place. They represent the only way we can get large doses of vitamins and supplements that may be needed. However, they cannot completely replace vitamins and minerals that occur naturally in raw fruits and vegetables. This is why I drink raw veggie juice everyday.

I was watching a vegetable juicer commercial on TV just the other day. The man doing the commercial was obviously very energetic and robust. He claimed to be 75 years old and credited his obvious good health to drinking fresh, raw vegetable juice daily. He said his favorite drink was carrot, beet, apple, and parsley. Coincidentally, that happens to be very similar to my drink.

Here is our exact recipe:

| 1 clove garlic | 1 stalk celery | 1/2 beet |
| 1/2 apple | 1 sprig parsley | 6 or more carrots |

Process the above in a juice extractor including enough carrots to make a total drink of 12 oz. Transfer to blender and add vitamins and supplements plus:

3 fresh or frozen strawberries

The juice from carrots and apples taste great. However, if you add many other ingredients, you can destroy the overall flavor. I have just discovered a way to make almost any vegetable drink taste excellent. By the way, just adding all the vitamins and supplements, to say nothing of the garlic, has a bad effect on the flavor. Make your vegetable juice in the normal manner. Pour the juice into a blender. Add all your supplements. Add two or three frozen strawberries. Alas, you have a drink that almost tastes like a strawberry milkshake. No, I'm not exaggerating. It really tastes great.

Colloidal Silver

This is another late update. Perhaps I need to explain what I mean by that. This book was finished sometime ago, or so I thought. It has not yet been accepted by a publisher, so I keep adding things that I learn about that I think are important. Colloidal Silver is one of them. Maybe I better explain what Colloidal Silver is. Colloid is a substance such as ultra-fine particles of silver suspended in an electrolyte such as distilled water. Colloidal Silver, more simply put, is distilled water containing very small particles of silver.

A friend of mine recently told me about his experience with Colloidal Silver. He and another friend of his both tried it and both had great improvement in their arthritic condition. I had no idea what it might do for me, other than help my arthritis, so I tried it. Much to my surprise, it speeded up the improvement in my ALS condition. I've been taking silver for about four months now. I have stopped taking the silver four times during the last four months and then restarted. Every time I stop and restart, I can recognize the effect of the silver. Therefore, I am convinced that it helps me. Additionally, my wife tried it on a very persistent skin rash on her arm and it caused immediate improvement, after other prescription drugs had failed.

Originally, I had no idea that it would help my ALS condition. That was a complete surprise. I began to wonder how it may have helped my ALS. I think I've figured it out. As you already know, I think that once you have ALS, then any and all toxins can adversely affect your condition. When I say toxins, that includes toxins caused by infection. At any given time, many of us may have minor infections in our bodies. They can occur in our urinary tract, our bowels, and our teeth and gums for instance. It is my belief that I must have some minor infection in my body and the silver has affected the infection and that resulted in an improvement.

According to what I read, Colloidal Silver has been known to successfully treat over 650 illnesses caused by bacteria, viruses, fungi, and parasites. One very important item about this strange mineral is that bacteria are unable to develop a resistance to it *and* there are no bad side effects. Here are only a few of the illnesses that have been successfully treated by Colloidal Silver:

Acne	Allergies
Arthritis	Cancer
Gonorrhea	Herpes
Lyme disease	Pneumonia
Psoriasis	Shingles
Syphilis	Warts

Now that, friends, is a pretty impressive list and this is only a small portion of them. I don't know if it is all true or not, but based on my own personal experience, I believe it could be. Here is a quote from an article published in *"Science Digest"* way back in March of 1978: "Thanks to eye-opening research, silver is emerging as a wonder of modern medicine. An antibiotic kills perhaps a half-dozen different disease organisms, but silver kills some 650. Resistant strains fail to develop. Moreover, silver is virtually non-toxic."

Apparently silver strengthens your immune system. Another great thing about silver is that it does not adversely affect your *good* bacteria. The bad bacteria have a negative charge and the silver is attracted to it because of its positive charge. Good bacteria, on the other hand, have a positive charge and the positive silver is not attracted to it.

Silver has been known to be of some help in preventing disease for over 1200 years. The Greeks and Romans used silver to line their eating and drinking utensils.

Prior to 1938, silver was the primary antibiotic treatment. Then, along came Penicillin and all the other more expensive and "modern" antibiotics and that was the end of silver.

I understand that you can buy Colloidal Silver at the health food store and it may come in various forms. However, the best and least expensive silver is a "do-it-yourself" project. If you are interested in making your own Colloidal Silver, there is a unit you can buy. It costs about $200 US.

The SilverGen SG6 Automatic colloid generator
Phone (877) 745-8374 or FAX (360) 732-5071

http://www.silvergen.com/General/order.htm

Creatine & Growth Hormone Booster

There are two supplements, which I have not included that you need to know about: Creatine and Growth Hormone Booster. The reason these are not listed earlier is because I had not taken them, as I had the others. Therefore, they have had no effect on my improvement. However, I have taken them off and on during the last several months and I think they both have great promise.

There's a great free report on Creatine on the Internet. Send an e-mail to the address below requesting a copy of the *"Creatine Answers for PALS"* report by Lynn Myers, MD:

Doctor@nucare.com

The doctor also provides a free weekly e-mail newsletter that covers various health and nutritional issues.

If you are interested in subscribing, just write "subscribe" in the subject line of your e-mail and send to:

Docjoc@nucare.com

Creatine and Vitamin E have both been proven effective on ALS in clinical trials according to what I read. There is much anecdotal evidence that Growth Hormone Booster is effective also. My problem is this. When I take either or both of these two products, I'm more inclined toward diarrhea. I've tried to take them several times, but had to quit. I seem to get almost instant improvement from Growth Hormone Booster. I believe both of these two items belong in our arsenal.

Sunshine

Sunshine may be just as important as any other supplement or vitamin. Don't worry about skin cancer. In spite of what some people say, the sun does not cause cancer. If it did, then all the Africans, Hawaiians, and Polynesians would be extinct. Actually, I believe that the sun creams cause skin cancer. After all they are just another toxin.

Sunshine is good for you. It creates Vitamin D and is essential for good health. However, be careful to not **burn**. Burning could contribute to skin cancer. Perhaps I'd better explain that some more. Toxins cause cancer. However, cancer can only get started in dead, dying or sick tissue. Sun burning the skin causes damage to the tissue and creates a great environment for cancer to get a start. If you suntan your skin slowly, you won't cause damage.

If you are out in the sunshine everyday for 30 minutes to an hour, you will probably never burn.

That's the end of my list of supplements.

In addition to taking a lot of supplements, there's one more thing that I do everyday. It is not exactly a supplement, but very important.

I take time everyday to pray and to think positive that I will improve. Glenna also reads several pages to me from the Bible every morning. Several times a day I will thank God for all that I have and ask Him to continue to show me the way. I also meditate several times each day about my improvement and concentrate on what still needs improving. I believe your body and your God have to know your program. They have to know what you want done and what your priorities are. They can only know this if you communicate with them everyday.

There's one other thing I do everyday. I read the comics in the newspaper. We all need a chuckle once in a while. The comics are not hilariously funny, but they're a lot more humorous than all the other stuff on the front page. There was a guy who wrote a book about curing a terminal disease by laughing. His prescription was to watch all the funny comedies and cartoons on TV. There are other books that have been written about what healing effect laughter can have on the human body.

Current Update – May 2002

I must bring you up-to-date on my latest supplement, which is Calcium with Vitamin D and Magnesium. I ran across a TV commercial not long ago about Calcium. They were interviewing a man who seemed to be most knowledgeable about Calcium. He seemed so credible in his statements that I ordered the product. Nothing ventured – nothing gained. I did not have high hopes for it, but I choose to leave no stone unturned. I received a two-month supply of Coral Calcium together with a book and a tape, both of which are extremely informative. The book is *"The Calcium Factor: The Scientific Secret of Health and Youth"* by Robert R. Barefoot and Carl J. Reich, MD.

Here is a website where you can order Barefoot's books:

http://www.calcium-factor.com/

Now here is something that you will find very interesting. It startled my wife. Included in the material is a pH test kit. Your pH can range from 4.5 to 7.5, 7.5 being desirable. My first test was 5.0. Then I thought, well maybe everyone is 5.0 so I had my wife test herself. She tested 7.5. Then I read more on the brochure under "Check Your Results." It said under #3 "If your pH is below 6.0, then you are highly acidic, very mineral deficient, and have contracted at least one degenerative disease."

Well, I don't have to tell you that caught my attention. I started taking 1000 units of the Coral Calcium daily. I noticed immediate improvement in my ability to move around. However, after about two weeks, I took another saliva test and although it was up some, it was still below 6.0. So, I doubled my intake to 2000 units a day. That was a week ago and I'm really impressed with my improvement. It is too early to really know, but I think this will be a real benefit and that's why I'm adding it now to the book. I just tested my saliva again and I'm now at 7.0 pH.

In the book *"The Calcium Factor,"* the authors tell us that Calcium or lack of it is the primary cause of many illnesses. I don't know if that's really true or not, because I think the root cause of many illnesses is toxins. However, I suppose it's possible that adequate Calcium could avoid the effect of toxins.

I would rather look upon Calcium as a Phase Two treatment but of course it may be a Phase One and Phase Two treatment; who knows? At any rate, I plan to be taking this Calcium for a long, long time.

Update – March 2004 – pH & Amalgams

I have read many articles about mercury and dental fillings called amalgams. This is one of the most controversial subjects ever discussed. People question why some people who have amalgam fillings don't have ALS or some other neurological condition.

It has been my pleasure to learn of something that might shed some light on that question. Dr. Robert Barefoot (the calcium doctor) claims that he had patients with mercury poisoning and the cause was their high-acid system and the acid was eating away their mercury amalgams.

I first heard about acid vs. alkaline in a book called *"Vermont Folklore Medicine"* written by a medical doctor. He claimed that many illnesses were directly caused by a person having a more acidic system and correction of that would or could possibly eliminate the illness. He recommended a diet of more alkaline food. Generally speaking, a vegetarian diet with less or no meat is more alkaline.

Edgar Cayce in his readings also discusses the need to correct your pH balance as a primary requisite for curing illness. If you don't know who he was, you may want to look at the following website:

http://hrrc@edgarcayce.org/

I also receive a monthly health newsletter written by a medical doctor. In a recent issue of his paper, he discussed the same thing about pH.

Now, back to the amalgams. This could explain why some people with amalgams have more illnesses than others with amalgams. Apparently, and quite possibly, if you have a low pH then you're transferring more mercury from your amalgams into your system.

I believe you can correct your pH imbalance by diet and/or a calcium supplement. My experience has been that you cannot correct your pH balance by calcium alone. Perhaps the following food list will help you:

Alkaline & Acidic Foods

Alkaline Foods (The higher the number, the more alkaline)

Group 1 – (+1 thru +6)
> Brussels sprouts +1, Asparagus +1, Lentils +1, Brazil nuts +1, Flax seeds +1, Olive oil +1, Buttermilk +1, Lettuce +2, Potato +2, Onion +3, Cauliflower +3, Tofu +3, Cabbage +4, Almonds +4, Flax seed oil +4, Peas +5, Sunflower seeds +5, Zucchini +6, Pumpkin +6

Group 2 – (+7 thru +14)
> Spinach +8, Lime +8, Lemon +10, Carrot +10, Green string beans +11, Red beets +11, Lima beans +12, Soy beans +12, White navy beans +12, Garlic +13, Celery +13, Cabbage lettuce +14, Tomato +14

Group 3 – (+15 or more)
> Avocado +16, Red radish +16, Soy nuts +26, Barley grass +29, Soy sprouts +30, Alfalfa grass +30, Cucumber fresh +32, Wheat grass +34, Soy lecithin +38, Black radish +39

> **Special note:**
> According to my own personal tests, bananas are highly alkaline although they are not on this list.

Acidic Foods (The higher the number, the more acidic)

Group 1 – (-1 thru – 6)
> Watermelon – 1, Homogenized milk – 1, Grapefruit – 2, Cantaloupe – 3, Liver – 3, Rye bread – 3, Cream – 4, Butter – 4, Strawberry – 5, Plum – 5, Whole-grain bread – 5

Group 2 – (-7 thru – 14)

>Sunflower oil – 7, Grape – 8, Walnuts – 8, Margarine – 8, Honey – 8, Papaya – 9, Orange – 9, Pear – 10, Peach – 10, Apricot – 10, Wheat – 10, White bread – 10, Cashews – 10, Fish, fresh water – 12, Ketchup – 12, Pineapple – 13, Brown rice-13, Mayonnaise – 13, Peanuts – 13

Group 3 – (-15 or more)

>Wine – 16, Cheese – 18, White sugar – 18, Mustard – 19, Fish, ocean – 20, Chicken – 20, Eggs – 20, Chocolate – 25, Coffee – 25, Beer – 27, Tea – 27, Liquor – 30, Fruit juice with sugar – 33, Beef – 34, Soy sauce – 36, Pork – 38, Vinegar – 39

These items are the most common foods and were obtained from a more comprehensive list.

The general idea here is not to eat only the alkaline foods. You want to reach a balance leaning toward alkaline food. To reach a healthy balance of 7.4 on your pH, you may only have to eliminate a few items with the higher numbers from the acidic list and add a few of the higher numbers on the alkaline list.

If you don't know your pH level, you can order a pH test kit by calling 1-800-899-8349.

Update – May 2004 – Important Note

Maybe I use too many words to write this book because many readers apparently overlook the importance of a major detox treatment. They seem to center on diet and supplements for one reason or another. That's why I am adding this important note.

There is no supplement known to me that is as effective as a detox treatment like DMPS chelation or Bentonite clay.

The only food that I know about that can be effective at eliminating mercury is cilantro.

CHAPTER 10

STARTING A NEW PROGRAM

I started my program in January '97. I was highly motivated to save my own life. Even though I have been successful with my program, I'm certain that very few PALS reading this book will actually adopt a program similar to mine. "Eric, that sounds strange. Why do you think that?" Well, I'll tell you. Two of the strongest forces in the universe are love and habit. These are two powerful forces and they are both invisible and sorely underestimated. *Habit* is the one we're concerned with here. By force of habit, you will do many of the same things today that you did yesterday. To change any of those habits is one of the most difficult tasks. The reason it is so difficult to change habits is because *you don't want to.* You like doing what you are doing or you wouldn't have created that habit in the first place. You might have a reason for *wanting* to break a habit. However, you probably really like doing it and you really *don't want to* change. That is the key. In order to change, you must *really want to* change.

Let's take smoking for example. Many people try to quit and fail. They know they should, but down deep, they really don't want to.

Knowing that habit is a powerful force, then we should be very careful about creating undesirable habits.

Here is a major universal cause of many of society's problems today.

Most people, upon reaching adulthood and moving out from under control of their parents, say to themselves, "I'm free at last. I can now do anything I want to do." And that, friends, is wrong thinking. There are universal rules for living in this world. To ignore them is man's greatest folly. I still remember what my Sergeant said in 1947 in the U.S. Army Basic Training. "You don't really have to do everything I tell you to do, but I guarantee you'll wish you had!" It is exactly the same with these universal rules. If you don't heed them, you will, sooner or later, wish you had. The late Gene Autry said upon reaching his 80th birthday, "If I had known I would live so long, I would have taken better care of my body."

There are rules of Mother Nature or God or rules of the universe; it doesn't matter what you call them, they exist. I'm going to call them "Universal Rules of Nature."

"Eric, what does all of this about universal rules have to do with my ALS?" Well, you probably have not been following these rules all your life and the reason I bring it up now is this. Now that you have ALS, you must start following the rules.

"Eric, what kind of rules are you talking about?" I mean things like over-eating, eating the wrong foods, drinking alcohol to excess, and failing to exercise, etc. If you eat too much of the wrong foods, you will get fat. That is a universal rule of nature. If you drink alcohol to excess, you will have health problems. That's another rule. Probably the number one rule is *stay close to nature*. If you have a choice between a natural product and a synthetic one, choose the natural product. An absolutely classic example occurred recently in my area. The *"Press Enterprise"* newspaper out of Riverside, California reported this story on the front page on 8-16-99. You might not believe this story, so I'm going to quote from the newspaper.

Headline

"BLIND, DYING TODDLER REBOUNDS AFTER
BEING FED BREAST MILK"

The story goes on to say, "For weeks, the 15-month-old had been sustained only by life-giving electrolytes" – "her body had rejected all other food and fluids."

Apparently the doctors and the family had given up all hope. The family had even purchased a coffin and made other plans accordingly. Then someone, other than the great medical doctors, suggested "Have you tried breast milk?" Two days after breast-feeding, the child was ready to come home. Two weeks later, her blindness was gone. What could be more *natural* than mother's milk? That is a remarkable story, but completely understandable. You see, the first thing they should have done, they did last: the first thing being the natural thing to do. Doctors, however, seldom consider *natural* treatments. They think they have all the answers they need in their drugs and surgery. Well this is one case where they were almost dead wrong. I repeat, stay as close to Mother Nature as possible

A second rule is – *take all things in moderation.*

This may be my most important rule. I have lived all of my life by this one. The middle of the road suits me just fine. I don't have to be the best at anything, but I'm not the worst either. A good example might be drinking alcohol. I've read about studies that indicate that a little bit of alcohol can actually be good for you. However, as you know, a lot can be very bad for you. Moderation is definitely the watchword when it comes to alcohol. Talking about alcohol, remember this rule.

If you drink, don't park. More people happen by accident!

I don't have a story about *moderation*, but I'm sure you get the message. There are exceptions to these rules and one such exception is in your treatment of ALS. That requires an all-out effort. If you're going to beat ALS, you better come out with both guns blazing. This is a matter of life and death. There's no room for moderation on this one.

I don't want to bring religion in here, but the Ten Commandments are examples of what I mean by universal rules of nature. Just like my Sergeant in the army said, "You don't have to follow the rules, but I guarantee you, if you don't, you'll wish you had." I will guarantee you that if you don't follow the Ten Commandments you will have a certain amount of chaos in your life. Look at Bill Clinton and his extramarital affairs. They are in direct violation of one of the Ten Commandments. Did he get away with it? At first blush you might think so. However, wouldn't you say his life has been just a little chaotic as a direct result of these affairs? Well, only if you call being impeached a little chaotic.

I don't mean to sound like a preacher right now, and I'm not perfect either, but I just want to make a point. You will see what I'm getting at in a moment. When I was in my early 20's, I realized these rules were there. Fortunately, my family taught me how to eat right and encouraged me to live a healthy lifestyle. I set rules for myself to follow. For example, I did not allow myself to drink alcohol at lunch time or for that matter anytime during the day until after work and after 5 PM. I think that's a good rule. I've seen friends of mine get in the *habit* of drinking two or three martinis everyday at lunch. They are all dead. Now I'm not here to tell you that I never had a drink before 5 PM. Yes, there were many times I did. But the point is they were exceptions for one reason or another. I never allowed myself to get in the *habit* of drinking that early.

"Well, hooray for you Eric. So what?" Well, the 'so what' is this; habits are hard to break and you may have to break many habits if you are to start a new program. Perhaps it was easier for me. I was already used to following my own rules. I am not reluctant to set new rules and/or change my habits. For example, I had enjoyed a glass of milk with every meal of everyday of my life until age 35. Let me tell you, that was a powerful *habit*. I thought I could not eat a meal without milk; totally impossible. Then, the doctor told me my cholesterol was way too high. I not only needed to lower my cholesterol, but I felt I had to and **wanted to.** Even though my milk drinking was a powerful *habit*, it was easy to break because I was already used to living by my own set of rules. Again, *habits* are easy to break if you *really want to.*

Since we're emphasizing the force of habits so much here, perhaps I should tell you about a procedure to help you break an old habit or create a new one. Let's say that you want to start a jogging program to improve your health. Here's what you do. Make the new task as easy as possible and then do it everyday that you have designated. For example, you want to jog everyday Monday through Friday only and you want to do it in the morning. You get up in the morning, jog down to the corner and back. That may sound too easy. However, you want to make it so easy that there's no excuse for not doing it. Next, you must do this every designated day for one month. If you skip one day, then you return to zero and start over until you have done it for one month. Now you can increase the distance but not too much. Do it in steps. I've done that on many things and it works quite well for me.

Now, let's look at another habit. This one is a real 'doozy.'

"Wait a minute, Eric; you keep using the word 'doozy.' I take it that means good, but what is the real meaning?" Well, in the 1930's, there was an automobile called a Duesenberg. It was the epitome of a first-class, sporty automobile. Many of the top movie stars of the day had one. 'Doozy' is short for Duesenberg. "That's a real doozy," became a very popular expression back then.

A real 'doozy' of a bad habit that probably 90% of us (including me) develop is coffee or coffee and a donut. I can sense that you are throwing rocks at me already. "Eric, why do you pick on coffee? I love it." I know. I loved it and still do. It was one of my toughest habits to break.

Coffee is a drug!

"Whoa, 'pardner,' you're getting carried away again." Well, let me explain. What is a drug? One definition of a drug is a substance that alters your mind or body; a stimulant or depressant. Coffee is unquestionably a stimulant. Everyone knows that, but we don't think of it as a drug; but it is. That's why it is so habit forming. Back to the universal rules of nature, one should not get into the habit of drinking coffee. If you drink a large amount of it everyday, it will sooner or later cause you a health problem. When I say sooner or later, I don't mean this as an absolute. We are all different and our tolerance for substance abuse varies from one to another.

Let me tell you about my experience with coffee. I used to have anxiety attacks quite often. They didn't know what they were in those days and they didn't have a name for it. I used to get shortness of breath, anxious feeling, nervous and I thought my chest would explode. Exercise would clear this up. One time I had a severe attack and decided to go immediately to my doctor. He gave me every test in the world including EKG, chest x-ray, etc. The only thing wrong was my blood pressure: 210 over 105! Wow, what could have caused that? Well, I really don't know, but coincidentally I had been at a meeting earlier that morning where I drank about ten cups of coffee. Incidentally, I had my blood pressure checked the next day and it was 118 over 78. I quit drinking coffee and started jogging Monday through Friday and I never had another anxiety attack. Depending on your tolerance for coffee, some of you might be able to get away with a cup or two a day. My experience would suggest that you limit your coffee. Of course, if you have a health problem, I would urge you to eliminate it entirely. Decaf is no substitute either. I would suggest green tea.

We are now back to January '97 and starting my program. If you have ALS or some other similar health problem, you may feel the need to start a program like mine. If you do not, I seriously urge you to stop reading right now and thoroughly analyze your otherwise hopeless situation. Encourage yourself to adopt your new health program. Recognize that if you don't change your eating habits and some other habits, you will probably not recover. Do you want to live and live an active life? If so, then it's within your power if you form some new habits.

Fortunately, it was easy for me to adopt my program. The timing was right, I was motivated by fear of death or total paralysis, and I was used to living by rules. I really wanted to live, and if that meant breaking many old habits, then that's simply what I had to do. It has now been seven years since I started it. I am immeasurably better than I was seven years ago. I'll give you more details in another chapter.

I enjoy a fairly comfortable lifestyle and continue to improve daily. I am pleased as punch that I started my program when I did. I know it requires a strong will to make a drastic change in your lifestyle. However, like Lawrence Taylor, pro-football player, said when he was being inducted into the Hall of Fame, "Anybody can quit. We all get knocked down at times. It's getting up that counts."

Starting a new program, and following it, is your goal. Like I said earlier, set your goal and work positively in the direction of your goal. If I can do it, you can do it. You simply have to have a strong desire to live.

CHAPTER 11

DRIVING A CAR

One of the most important things that you must do, once you realize you have ALS, is to maintain as much physical activity as possible. If you don't, your muscles will waste away sooner and you will develop limited range of motion much faster. Getting into and out of the car and driving a car is an activity that you should keep up as long as possible. Now, don't get me wrong. If you become an unsafe driver, then you should quit immediately. However, *you* are the best judge of that. With all that in mind, let me tell you my story.

I continued driving long past my crisis point when I was in my worse physical condition. Why? Because I was still capable of driving and I wanted to maintain that activity. Even my wife had absolutely no complaints about my driving ability. But, a strange thing happened. People, (shall I call them "friends?") began to tell my wife behind my back that she should not let me drive. None of these so-called friends had ever ridden with me and so could not even begin to evaluate my driving ability. However, they set themselves up as experts on driving with ALS. So many people did this, that finally my wife caved in. She asked me not to drive and she was very insistent. Well, I gave up driving rather than fight with her. However, as I look back, that was a big mistake. During the six months that I did not drive, my driving ability deteriorated only from limited range of motion. To make a long story short, I have since been tested by the California Department of Motor

Vehicles twice. One time was a driving test only and I passed the test with flying colors. The second time, they gave me a written test, driving test and eye test. I missed one question on the written, the eye test was perfect as I have 20/20 vision in both eyes, and again I passed the driving test with flying colors. Most people don't understand that ALS is *selective* in the muscles effected. For example, in my case, I can't walk without the aid of a walker, but my feet work quite well on the gas and brake pedals. The problem with driving when you have a disability is really mental. You must make mental adjustments based on your driving ability. For example, the younger drivers, age group 16 to 25, are the most physically capable drivers of any age group. However, they have the worst driving record. They have more accidents by more than 2 to 1 compared to all other age groups. The reason is simple; they drive beyond their capability. Conversely, when you have a disability, you must learn to drive *within* your capability.

The point of all this is, "Don't let this happen to you." Don't let others tell you what to do. I must say one more time, however, that you should continue driving *only* as long as you are *capable*.

The real message that I want to get across here is this: Virtually everyone has a strong prejudice against handicapped drivers. When they find out you have ALS, they immediately jump to the conclusion that you should not be driving. I thought my friends and family would be glad to hear that I was still *capable* of driving. However, they don't see it that way. My only purpose in writing this chapter is to forewarn. To be forewarned is to be forearmed. Enough said.

CHAPTER 12

MY ALS SYMPTOMS

You have heard my story from the beginning up to January 1997 when I started my program. We will now continue from there.

There was a period when my system continued to get worse even though I was on my program. There was about a two-month overlap. I started the day after Thanksgiving '96. However, I wasn't into all phases until January '97. I continued to get worse until around March of '97. By April and May of '97, I had realized nothing was worse and a few things were improving. Most noticeable was my choking. That began to improve. I wasn't choking as often. I continued to improve for the next few months, but then I had hip surgery in July '97 and that slowed me down a little. Toward the end of '97, I began learning more and more about amalgam dental fillings. I finally became convinced that they had to be removed. However, I didn't find the right dentist until March '98. Prior to March '98, a strange thing was taking place. I was improving in all areas, except my left arm. My left arm was going downhill. Muscle atrophy and paralysis was setting in. It is strange how I can improve in one area and get worse in another. I don't quite understand it, but that's what happened.

Shortly after removal of my amalgams, my left arm began to improve. It has been getting stronger ever since. More on this later. Another strange thing happened at this same time. I told you I had severe arthritis in my left shoulder. You may not believe this, but after the amalgam removal, my left shoulder began to improve also. What a pleasant surprise that was. I really did not expect that to happen.

Almost any medical doctor will, upon hearing or reading of my success with ALS, immediately question whether or not I really had ALS. I've heard this many times. Apparently most MD's think there is no cure for ALS. So, if you get better, then you **must not have had ALS**. Well, that's pretty narrow-minded and another example of a pre-established belief that needs to be challenged. I recognize that their narrow-mindedness does exist. Actually, any reasonable person should question this of course.

With that in mind, let me tell you of all my symptoms and at the same time how they improved.

I believe I have had all the classic symptoms of ALS and, of equal importance, I have no other symptoms that might indicate a different illness. For example, MS people cannot tolerate heat. I have no problem with heat. Most ALS patients have normal mental ability. I think I have had no deterioration in my mental ability. It is quite the contrary; my mental ability has improved. It is typical for PALS to have normal sexual function. I have suffered no deterioration in that department. Yeah, yeah, yeah . . . . so what?

Now let's review each of my symptoms:

Muscle Weakness

Muscle weakness is the primary problem with ALS. I had it almost everywhere. I had lost strength in both hands and arms, both legs, and my torso including stomach, back, and neck.

I also had loss of muscle control in my mouth and throat affecting my swallowing. There was a time when I was choking two or three times a day. I've had a choking problem since I was 18 years old. However, it would occur very infrequently. With the onset of ALS and the difficulty in swallowing, the choking problem became far more frequent. If I swallowed wrong and something got anywhere near my windpipe; my throat muscles would involuntarily clamp shut. When this would happen, I could not breathe in the least. This would scare poor Glenna to death. It never worried me too much, because I knew in about 30 or 40 seconds, I would be able to breathe slightly and within five minutes be normal again. This was never life threatening, but certainly not a fun experience.

My speaking was also affected. I have to speak more slowly and more deliberately to be understood. If I get lazy, you can't understand me. Other than breathing and swallowing, I value the ability to speak more than any other muscle function. I am fortunate that my speaking ability never deteriorated to the point that I could not be understood with proper effort.

I don't believe muscle weakness ever affected my breathing. I have had breathing tests that indicated around 90%. Well, that *ain't* bad for an old duffer like me!

Muscle Atrophy

I had severe muscle atrophy in both forearms and both upper arms. I had mild atrophy in my legs and torso.

Weight Loss

As your muscles get weaker and atrophy sets in, you naturally lose a lot of weight. In a short time, in the fall of '96, I lost about 20 pounds. I went from almost 160 down to well under 140. My lowest weight ever was 136.

Muscle Fasciculations

Yes, I had these too but they are of no consequence. There is no pain or discomfort. The doctor described them as being like worms crawling under your skin. Actually, they're just little twitches in the muscles.

Muscle Cramps

As you probably know, muscle cramps are painful. That's when the muscle contracts way beyond the normal contraction. I had these frequently for a while. These would usually occur in the morning. That's when you wake up and need to stretch a lot. Every time I would stretch my legs way out, the stretch would turn into a muscle cramp.

Muscle Spasms

Spasms are similar to cramps and sometimes precede cramps, but spasms are not really painful. Spasms are where the muscle involuntarily contracts but within its normal range. I get spasms in my legs every morning when I stretch.

Muscle Stiffness

Maintaining range of motion is very important to a PALS. I did not do this the way I should have and I developed a lot of stiffness in my legs. I should have continued an exercise program involving maximum leg motion. When I say stiffness I mean just like rigor mortis sets in. I can't move my legs beyond a certain point and no one else can move them for me.

Coordination & Balance

When the muscles get weak, they also fail to respond quickly. This problem was most noticeable to me when I could still walk without the aid of a walker. I would fall down frequently by just stubbing my toe on the least little thing. I could not move my legs quickly enough to recover. I would lose my balance easily. It seems that my body would lean more before I realized it. This made it easy to fall down.

Lack of muscle coordination is most apparent in swallowing. Swallowing is an almost automatic procedure. You don't normally think about it. With ALS, however, swallowing is difficult because it involves the careful coordination of the tongue, the esophagus and other muscles of the throat.

Fatigue

You know all about this one. Fatigue is what you feel at the end of the day. The difference with PALS and with me is, when I get up in the morning, I feel like it is at the end of the day.

Cold Sensitivity

I really had cold sensitivity. I could hardly stand to be all wet after showering. I had to be dried off as quickly as possible. I can't explain it exactly, but somehow the cold affects the nerves.

One time I sat in the swimming pool for over an hour. The water was heated and seemed warm enough. However, it evidently wasn't warm enough. When I went to get out, I could not move my legs due to the cold. They just wouldn't work. Two men had to lift me out of the pool.

I read about another PALS who wound up in the hospital from eating a Popsicle. He had a seizure brought on by the sudden cold of the Popsicle.

Bowels

I have read that ALS does not normally affect the bowels. I don't believe that. I have talked to many other PALS who have bowel problems. It is simple to understand. The weaker muscles make it difficult to have a BM. By the same token, the weaker muscles make it difficult to not have a BM. In other words, it's real easy to "mess your drawers." I did this frequently for a time. The worse one occurred in my recliner. It was everywhere. Half of it in my chair, half of it on the carpeting, and the residue was in my shorts and running down my legs. This is one of the worst times for a caregiver like my wife, Glenna. Glenna says "Amen, brother, Amen! An event like that is enough to make you want to leave home." After that, I wore diapers for a while.

Emotions

My emotions became very acute. Both crying and laughing were more extreme. This is both strange and funny at the same time. I've always been a pretty good storyteller. I love to tell dirty jokes about men, women, and sex and all that stuff. ALS gave me a real problem though. When I tried to tell a funny story, I would start laughing so hard I couldn't talk before I got to the punch line. I had to give up storytelling for a while.

Speaking of storytelling, it's about time for a story. We have an all-black cat named Sabrina. She has a really cute trick. In the morning, I read the newspaper. It is delivered folded up with a rubber band around it. I remove the rubber band and place it on the kitchen table next to me. (By the way, I can hold the newspaper in my right hand, and remove the rubber band with my left hand. There was a time when that was impossible.) Sooner or later, Sabrina will appear at my right side. She will stand up on her hind legs and with her right front paw, reach up and scoop the rubber band off of the table. She will play with it, throw it up in the air, and have a great time for a while. When she gets bored with it, she'll put it in her food dish. I don't know why she does that. Lately, however, she has taken to eating the rubber band. Glenna told me that Sabrina was not feeling well lately and apparently not eating. I said to Glenna, "Don't worry, she will *snap back!*" There was only one problem; I was laughing so hard at my own joke that I couldn't get out the words "snap back."

The other side of the coin, crying, was more of a problem. I would cry at the drop of a hat. When I cried, it wasn't sobbing, it was extreme. Prior to ALS, I never cried more than a half a dozen times in my whole life. I mean it, I just never cried, period. I've told you that we used to make frequent weekend dune buggy trips in the desert. As a result, there was a great deal of maintenance necessary, such as mechanical adjustments, repairs, and oil changes, etc. I used to do most of that myself. I got to know the layout at Pep Boys pretty well as I went there often for supplies and parts. One day we were driving through the parking lot of a large shopping center. I looked over and saw the Pep Boys sign. I immediately went into a severe crying jag. These used to scare the pants off Glenna. Most anything sad would set me off. Boy, I'm glad I don't do that anymore.

Love, Sex and the ALS Patient

I pondered and pondered about including this, but I must. To exclude this subject from any discussion of ALS would be a serious oversight.

Many people don't like to discuss sex. However, sex is a fundamental part of life. If it weren't for sex, you would not exist. Neither would I. Sex is to love, like nectar is to honey. Like a mountain stream feeds a lake and keeps it alive, sex nourishes love. Sex enhances love and love enhances a relationship. Sex is the most loving and intimate act that ever occurs with two people. Now, here's the problem.

The problem with many ALS patients is their body muscles are partially or totally paralyzed while their brain and sex drive remains normal. Probably dementia and/or impotence, along with ALS, would be a blessing in disguise. I am speaking from a man's point of view.

The ALS patient loses his ability to move about physically in the normal lovemaking process early in his deterioration. This all becomes very "un-macho" as he loses his ability to seduce. Where does that leave him?

Can you imagine, for just a moment, being totally paralyzed and having an itch on your forehead? That is a mild torture. If you could only ask someone to scratch your forehead for you, wow, what a relief that would be.

If the PALS has a spouse or a lover, perhaps they can help.

Sleep

A sleeping problem may not be a direct symptom of ALS. However, it seems to be a universal problem of all handicapped people. Or should I have said physically challenged? No, that's not for me. I consider myself physically handicapped. A spade is a spade!

There is no doubt that the cause of your sleep problem is the lack of exercise. There is probably not much you can do about that. I had quite a problem with sleeping for a while. Then I learned a couple of things that helped me a great deal.

First, do not sleep for more than 20 minutes at a time during the day.

Second, get up every morning at precisely the same time. This may require you to go to bed at the same time also, but that is not as important.

Third, relocate to a chair or some other location during the day when you're normally awake. Take your naps there too, if you can. This tells your body that when you go to bed you're there to sleep.

This may not sound like much, but if you will do it I guarantee you will be able to sleep better. It will take about ten days to two weeks to establish a new sleeping regimen. I was having a great deal of trouble getting to sleep at night. Sometimes it would take two or three hours. Occasionally I would still be awake at 3:00 or 4:00 AM. I normally go to sleep within fifteen minutes. I watch TV in my recliner chair until 11:00 PM. I go to bed then, and I'm asleep by 11:30. I wake up at 7:30 AM and I am out of bed by 8:00 AM. I follow this schedule seven days a week.

Well folks, there they are. Those are all my symptoms. To the best of my knowledge, which comes from discussions with MD's, neurologists and many PALS, these are typical for all PALS. Again, I want to point out that these are my *only* symptoms. I do not have any other symptoms or any other health problem other than arthritis in my left shoulder. I have 20/20 eyesight. My blood pressure ranges around 110 over 75. It never varies more than about five points in either direction. I feel great. I suffer no pain. I have no numbness. I have no indication of dementia. I am probably the healthiest man you would ever meet with a terminal disease. I am certain that I have stopped the progress of ALS to the extent that I can reasonably say that I no longer have ALS. However, like the victim of polio, I still have the effects of the damage caused by ALS.

I have tried to illustrate all of these symptoms in depth. The reason is to convince you that I had ALS. As I said before, too many people want to say I never had ALS and chalk up my recovery to misdiagnosis in the beginning. In my mind, there are no two ways about it. I had ALS. I had all the symptoms and all the tests. All the tests proved negative for any other disease or health problem. Four different neurologists have diagnosed me and they all agreed on ALS as my problem.

In the next chapter, I will tell you about my progress and how many of these symptoms have improved.

CHAPTER 13

THE ALS COMEBACK

Now I will attempt to bring you up-to-date on all of my improvements. This way, you can be the judge on the success of my program.

Muscle Strength – Arms & Legs

My very first symptom of ALS, which occurred way back in '91, was in my right hand. I first noticed it when I would attempt to close the heavy drapes by pulling on the thin drapery cord. My fingers weren't strong enough to hold on while I pulled the cord. It progressed very slowly at first. Eventually, however, my right arm and hand became almost useless. It would work some, but I wouldn't dare pick up a glass and attempt to lift it to my mouth. The few times I tried it, I failed. I would drop the glass about half way up. I could eat food with a fork in my right hand if I was very careful. However, I could not cut a pancake with a fork in my right hand. I am right-handed so I would normally hold my electric razor in my right hand to shave. My right hand and arm got so weak I couldn't hold the razor. I had to put the razor in my right hand, and then wrap my left hand around my right hand and the razor, and shave that way.

Oddly enough, my right hand began improving way back around 1994. Many other muscle groups deteriorated since then, but my right hand and arm has continued to improve. Today, my right hand and arm is about 80% of what it was before ALS. It is strong enough to do most anything I want to. I don't have normal dexterity with my fingers. For example, it is difficult to deal cards. That's pretty good though, everybody else has to deal for me. How good can it get?

My right leg was the second limb to be affected. We were at a Christmas party dance in '92. I was sitting at a table attempting to move my right leg up and down with the beat of the music. I realized that I couldn't move it quickly enough to stay in time with the music. This is when I first realized that I had a really serious problem. It really frightened me. Whatever the problem, it had spread from my right arm to my right leg. Eventually my right foot became very weak. I noticed this when driving the car. If I only put the ball of my foot on the brake pedal, I didn't have strength enough to press on it. I had to be very careful to get more of my heel on the brake pedal. Eventually, my right ankle became stiff and would not bend at all. Fortunately, I had an automatic transmission car and could easily brake with my left foot. I had driven that way most of my life anyway.

Today, my right ankle has normal flexibility and my right foot has about 90% of the strength I had originally.

Somewhere around 1996, my ALS moved into my left leg and left arm. It never affected my left leg that much. To this day, my left leg is very near normal.

At one time, when I would stretch my legs out while lying down, my feet would cross. I could do nothing to avoid them crossing. That no longer occurs. I can stretch my legs out with my feet parallel to each other and even turn the feet out.

My left arm is another story. My left arm deteriorated to the point that I had no grip in my left hand. Also, I could move my arm very little. I had to move my left arm by grabbing it with my right hand and placing it where I wanted it. I could still drive a car, but turning was difficult because of my left arm. It was extremely difficult to lift my left arm high enough to reach the turn indicator lever in my car. I had extreme pain in my left shoulder and my arm movements were very awkward and uncoordinated. Well, about this time, I gave up driving for a while.

I should mention one point about the use of my arms. I was very fortunate that both arms were never paralyzed at the same time. I say fortunate because I was always able to use one arm or the other to pick my nose, wipe my butt, and perform other important functions. My right hand was the first to go. I always was a little ambidextrous, so I was able to switch and use my left hand. Then by the time my left hand and arm became paralyzed, my right one was working again.

Today I have adequate strength in my left hand to grip and to hold most anything. I can raise my left arm to the turn indicator in the car with no pain. I can move my left arm in all directions except not beyond shoulder height. However, that's the arthritis in the shoulder causing that. When you're eating soup, and you get near the bottom, you tip the bowl so you can spoon out all of it. Well, I absolutely could not and would not dare to do that with my left hand. Now I can and I haven't spilled yet.

Some of these improvements are certainly not earth shaking. You must realize, however, that the medical doctors say it's impossible. Any improvement at all feeds my Positive Mental Attitude like pouring gas on a fire. Obviously, the slightest improvement means a great deal to me and I know there is more to come.

Muscle Strength – Torso

At one time, my overall body strength was minimal. When I sat down on the edge of the bed, I didn't lie down, I fell down. Glenna would have to pick up my legs and move them up and onto the bed at the same time my torso fell back onto the bed. Once I was lying down on my back, I was pretty much immobile. The only way I could turn on my side was by grabbing the edge of the bed with my hand and pulling my body over. When Glenna dressed me, she had to lift each leg to slip my pants on. Then she had to roll me from side to side to pull my pants all the way up to my waist. When I was lying down on my back in bed, I could barely raise my head off the pillow.

Today I can sit on the bed, roll onto my back, pull my knees up high enough to clear the edge of the bed, and lay down without any help. I can roll over onto my side without grabbing or pulling on anything. I can lift my head off the pillow and I can raise my head and shoulders up several inches off the bed. In other words, I can do about a half of a sit up. Again, when lying on my back, I can lift each leg separately up in the air and hold it there while Glenna puts my pants on. That means holding your legs up in the air parallel to the bed. That's actually a pretty good trick for someone who never had ALS. That is a real improvement. When she gets my pants half on, I raise my knees and pull my feet up close to my butt. I can then lift my entire butt and back off of the bed so Glenna can pull my pants up to my waist. That's another real improvement.

Glenna and I recently went to Laughlin, Nevada. That's the 'Poor Man's' Las Vegas. We stayed at Harrah's Hotel and had a nice room, but we forgot to bring a support bar for the bed. Since I didn't have one, I was forced to improvise. From lying on my back in bed, I was able to move into a sitting position on the edge of the bed without any help and without pulling on any support. It was difficult, but I did it. I had not been able to do that for over two years. I am making progress although it seems very slow at times.

Current Update – March 2002

I simply must add this note on what my muscles are doing now. Have you ever exercised more than normal and then wake up the next morning with stiff and sore muscles? When that happens that means that your muscles are growing. Well, for several months now, I have been waking up with stiff and sore muscles as though I had a really heavy workout the day before. Sore may not be the right word because the feeling is a good one. I feel healthy and stronger. My muscles are firm and growing. This is more than ever before. I'm just absolutely certain that I will restore my body to the same level as before in time.

Atrophy & Weight Loss

I had a lot of muscle atrophy in both arms. I have regained about half of the muscle that I lost. At one time, the muscles were thin and hung from my bones like wet long-john underwear on the clothesline. Now they have firmed up considerably.

My legs never atrophied much at all. They are fairly normal.

At one time, I had lost around 20 pounds, which was muscle and fat. When I first regained about 15 pounds, it was some muscle but a lot of fat. I have since lost about 10 pounds of fat. I need to add a little more muscle but my fat is minimal, where it should be.

Walking

Let me tell you about a blessing in disguise that occurred during my deterioration period. Way back in the early stages of my ALS symptoms, around '91 and '92, I had a problem that I will call anxious legs. This would occur when I would go to bed at night. My legs would get this anxious feeling where I just had to move them. Usually, after two or three hours of thrashing around, I would sit up on the edge of the bed. Having nothing else to do at 1:00 or 2:00 AM, I would stand up with my walker and do deep knee bends. Well, maybe not really *deep*, but knee bends just the same. Actually, I would do about a 3/4 knee bend. This helped me maintain muscle strength in my legs and avoided muscle atrophy. I actually did this exercise almost every night for several years. If it wasn't for my 'anxious-legs' problem, I probably would not have done the knee bends as frequently as I did. That's why I say the 'anxious-legs' problem was really a blessing in disguise.

Based on my experience with ALS and particularly as the above illustrates, I would strongly recommend that you maintain all physical movement possible by doing all the exercises you are capable of doing. Do not quit doing anything because it is difficult. Keep doing it as long as you can. Remember, an ounce of prevention is worth a pound of cure.

Today both legs appear quite normal and they are very strong. I would probably be able to walk quite normally if it wasn't for two things. First, I had hip replacement surgery in my left hip in July '95 and right hip July '97. After hip replacement surgery, they have you walking in one or two days. Walking however is limited to short steps. As a result, rigor mortis set in and I am now unable to take long steps. Second, for a month or two prior to my right hip replacement, I was walking with a cane and leaning way over to my right and forward. Again, rigor mortis set in and even after hip replacement I could not stand up straight. Not only that, I couldn't sit up straight in a firm chair. You see, my back was bent to the right so much that the right butt bone was pulled way up. I'm not fat, so when I sit on a hard surface, I'm normally sitting directly on my two butt bones. This irregularity required that I sit in a chair with arms. Otherwise, I would fall over and fall right out of the chair. I have been working on my back for about two years. I even went to the hospital for physical therapy which didn't help much. I just continue everyday to bend my back to the left as far as possible and as often as I think about it. It's working, but very slow. This makes it impossible to walk normally because when I step on my left leg, my upper body weight is way over to the right. I have made a lot of progress. Now I can sit in a chair or on the toilet without fear of falling off. My walking is improving as my weight becomes more centered. When I eventually get my back straight, I'm sure I'll be chasing Glenna around the bedroom again.

I really only have two problems today related to ALS: walking and talking. If those would improve just a little bit more, I could not ask for more. I could live the rest of my days quite comfortably without any complaint.

Talking

If you would have heard me talk back in January '97 and then hear me today, you would say there is no improvement. However, there has been a lot of change in the muscles of my tongue, throat and mouth. It hasn't improved my speech yet, but I'm confident it will. It's only a matter of time. Right now, I am dictating this to my wife, Glenna, who is typing on the computer. I speak slowly but I rarely have to repeat myself. I can speak quite clearly if I speak loud and forcefully.

Update – December 2000

At long last, I finally have noticeable improvement in my speech. It isn't much and it varies from time to time. Nonetheless, improvement is improvement and I'm certain that the improvement will continue.

Muscle Fasciculations

I still have some muscle twitching but very minimal. This is actually a good sign, I think, because it means they are still alive and kicking.

Muscle Cramps

I haven't had a muscle cramp for several months.

Muscle Spasms

I still have spasms in my legs when I stretch my legs out after they have been bent at the knee for a while.

Muscle Stiffness

I still have muscle stiffness in my lower back and in my legs. It is improving in both areas. However, the improvement is very slow. When I step onto my electric cart, my step is measurable. I can reach my foot further into the electric cart by several inches. The only way I can tell about my back is by visual observation and the fact that my weight is more centered.

Coordination & Balance

Coordination and balance have both improved. I see improvement in my coordination in turning the pages of the newspaper. It used to be very awkward. I'm now much better at it. Improvement in my balance is evidenced by my ability to free-stand for as long as a half a minute without holding on to anything.

Fatigue

I used to be tired all the time. If we went for even a short ride in the car, I would fall asleep every time. I don't have that problem anymore. I feel energetic now.

Cold Sensitivity

My sensitivity to cold is almost normal now. When I'm wet after showering, I don't have that cold feeling anymore. When I move from the car to the house on a cold evening, I do not get the horrible chilled feeling I used to get. What a great improvement that is.

Bowels

This is still a problem. I have it under control so I no longer wear diapers and I rarely have an accident. In fact, I've now gone five months without an accident. However, I use an enema daily. The gut muscles just won't work on their own without some priming. At least I'm not messing my drawers so that's an improvement. Glenna says "Amen, brother, Amen!"

Emotions

I haven't cried in many months. Boy, am I glad of that. That was horrible. However, my laughing is about the same, but I can certainly live with that. How could I complain about laughing too much? It just means that my audience has to be more patient and wait for the punch line (I'm laughing now as I dictate this to Glenna).

General Health

My general health is excellent. I have normal blood pressure and no abnormality in my blood or urine. I am very healthy. I have no pain and I feel great. My friends are always asking me how I feel. Well, my answer is "I feel fine, and I always have." I simply have restricted use of my legs and some other minor problems listed above.

As I view my progress today, I think it is important to consider the treatment of ALS as a *two-phase* program.

Phase One of my treatment program was developed with one primary goal: *Stop the progress of ALS.* There is absolutely no doubt in my mind, or that of any doctor that has seen me, that I have accomplished that goal. Phase Two is to *improve my physical condition.* I am clearly in Phase Two now. There is no point attempting to rebuild muscles until you have stopped the progress of ALS. I have recently found a new doctor to help me with this phase (Dr. Rouzier). He works with chelation, hormone therapy, etc. This new doctor gave me a thorough blood and urine laboratory checkup recently and told me "You are physically perfect on paper."

Every single item in the lab report was in a near perfect range, such as, thyroid, cholesterol, triglycerides, all three electrolytes, glucose, liver, and many, many more. Apparently my diet and supplement program must be having some good affect on my health. Remember I'm 72 years old!

I have been working with the doctor about six months and I'm getting great results. Before I started on this program, I could only do about 20 or 30 knee bends at one time. When I say knee bends, I mean about a two-thirds of a knee bend. Recently, I have done as many as 105 knee bends at one time. Now that is real measured improvement. I clearly feel stronger in all of my body. My muscles appear to be firmer and some muscles have *actually grown!* I began measuring my arms, legs, waist and chest about three months ago. Since then, I have added ¾ of an inch to each arm. Additionally, I have gained five pounds (and it *ain't* fat). I plan to continue on my current program of hormone therapy and vitamin/mineral IV. Incidentally, this IV includes *restorative* ingredients such as Glutathione.

I like to tell people, when they ask about my health, "I'm probably the healthiest person you will ever meet with a so-called *terminal illness.*"

I have told you of every improvement. Like a friend of mine used to say, "I'm in pretty good shape, for the shape I'm in!"

Update – December 2001

It has now been over eighteen months that I've been seeing Dr. Rouzier and continuing my vitamin/mineral IV with Glutathione. Additionally, I have a shot of testosterone at every visit, which is every two to four weeks. My rate of improvement has increased. I feel stronger than ever. Recently I did 200 knee bends at one time. I started curling a five-pound dumb bell with each arm. Previously, I could not do a single curl with my left arm. I've only been doing this a few weeks now and I'm up to fifty curls with each arm.

My talking has greatly improved lately. It still varies from day to day and I don't know why. Glenna cannot see much difference, but I can tell when it's much easier to put words closer together than before. A year ago, I could not even begin to sing a song, because I could not transfer from one word to the other fast enough to keep up with the tune. I can now although I still have trouble hitting the notes correctly. At any rate, there has been much improvement.

CHAPTER 14

DOING IT OVER

It has occurred to me that you might be wondering what I would do if I were starting all over again. Obviously I've learned a lot since I began my program and, therefore, I would not do everything exactly the same. For example I did not have my amalgams removed until two years after I began my program. Also, I did not start chelation until three and one-half years after.

Sometimes I think I used too many words to write this book, and I worry that the fundamentals may be overlooked by some readers. That's what this chapter is all about. It occurred to me that an outline of my regimen might be a good idea so I created one. You will find the outline included in the back of this book. You may want to remove it for ready reference.

Before we continue though, I simply must tell you a story. By now you know that I love to tell stories, particularly if they have meaning. This one has meaning.

In the beginning of my great ALS experience I began to pray frequently. My prayer at that time went something like this: "God, thank you for all that I have and help me find the way to treat or cure this terrible disease." About a year ago I changed my prayer and my new prayer went something like this: "God, thank you for all that I have and all of my progress. However, I really must ask you for more help. I've been improving for seven years and you have certainly been instrumental in my improvement. I sincerely believe that I have suffered long enough and hard enough. Could you please help me speed up my recovery? I will be forever grateful and will endeavor to help others more."

Within just a few short months of my new prayer, information about ALS treatments that were all new to me began coming to me from various sources. I have learned of more new treatments in the last few months than for any similar previous time period.

Now you can chalk that up to coincidence if you want to. However, as I said before, if you believe in coincidence you will not make a very good detective.

All of these new treatments caused me to completely reorganize my regimen outline. For example: I thought previously that some form of detox treatment should be the first item. However, now I have learned that if you have any amalgams, they should be removed first because your body may not detox as well if the amalgams are still in your system. Therefore, amalgam removal must be first before detox. Additionally, you may not want to do any detox treatments until after all the amalgams have been removed. Amalgam removal alone will put enough burden on your system.

Here is another thought. Depending on how far advanced your ALS condition is and/or depending on your overall health, you may want to improve your condition prior to either amalgam removal or detox. You may want to begin a nutritious diet and supplement program. Also, if you have constipation or diarrhea, perhaps you should improve your digestive system to eliminate either of those problems. You must have a digestive system in good working order before you do any detox treatment.

This should explain why I have revised the order of the things I would do. I would do diet and supplements first for a time, amalgam removal next, and one or more detox treatments to follow.

Please refer to my outline at the end of this book for more details.

Hopefully, some of you who are reading this book do *not* have ALS or some similar disorder. This portion of the book is for you as well as a PALS.

When you're first born into this world you pretty much accept things the way they are. However, you hear older people talking about problems and that some things are going from bad to worse. If you have a positive mental attitude, you will tend to ignore them. I was like that. I had to live to be over sixty years old to discover and fully realize that we have some very serious threats to our health right here in the good old U.S. of A. For the past six or seven years, I have been focused on these threats and I have read many articles and books on this subject. My conclusion is that we not only have a serious problem, it is of *epidemic* proportions. Now, I'm not exaggerating when I say *epidemic.* If we have a problem that faces the majority of the people living in this country, wouldn't you consider that an epidemic? Well, that's exactly what we have. I could give you a lot of statistics, but all you have to do is read the obituaries for several days and draw your own conclusions. You will find very few people die of natural causes. You will find that over 90% die of cancer, heart problems, AIDS, and several chronic illnesses like ALS. Even though these people may have been 70 or 80 years old when they died, they would have lived longer without the cancer, etc. So what's the point? The point is they are all *preventable.* Most of these illnesses, including cancer and excluding heart to some degree, are caused by toxins. If we were not exposed to the toxins, then we would not have most of these illnesses.

Now, think about that for just a minute. Ninety percent or more of the people dying in this country nowadays are dying from a *preventable illness.* I think that is terrible and unacceptable. The problem is further aggravated by the fact that most people are not aware of this.

Remember that I'm talking to you people who are healthy now.

Warning

You are living in the most polluted environment since pollution wiped out the dinosaurs millions of years ago. You may already know that, but what are you doing about it? Here is my urgent suggestion for all healthy people reading this.

Do something to **detoxify** your body before it's too late. An ounce of prevention is worth a pound of cure. When it comes to our health, I believe an ounce of prevention is worth **five** pounds of cure.

Most mammals live to be seven times their age at maturity. For example, a horse matures around the age of three *and* they live to be twenty years or even much more. I had a horse that lived to be 37 years old. I bought the horse for my daughter when the horse was twelve. So I'm pretty sure of the age when he died. That would be like a man living to be about 300 years old.

Based on the multiple of seven rule, people should live to be around 130 or 140. Now that's a far cry from the average life expectancy today. At any rate, that should provide you with further evidence that 90% of us are dying prematurely.

If I could go back to a time *before* I had my first ALS symptom, what would I do differently? That's easy. I would do all the things I already told you about only I wouldn't go to the *extreme*. I would have my amalgams removed without any question. I would do chelation and other detox treatments. I would try to follow a good diet about 80 or 90% of the time. Again, I'm not normally an extremist and I don't think you have to be.

I would begin by taking at least the following supplements:

Multi-Vitamin and Minerals
Co-enzyme Q-10
Alpha-lipoic acid
Vitamin B Complex
Vitamin C
Vitamin E
Vitamin A
DHEA
Colloidal Silver
Calcium including Vitamin D and Magnesium

One last thought. Alzheimer's is a preventable illness and again, I believe caused by toxins. They say that 50% of us who live to be 85 will have Alzheimer's. Now that folks is an epidemic all by itself.

Paul Bragge wrote several books on the effects of toxins and good health. I read one of his books over thirty years ago. If I would have done even some of the things that he suggested doing, I believe I would not have ALS today.

Even the Bible tells us to treat our body as a temple. Keep it pure and pristine. Maintaining good health is an obligation you have not only to yourself, but also to your immediate family and loved ones.

I realize that the things I'm talking about doing are all preventative treatments and are not covered by insurance. Therefore, you will have to pay for these treatments yourself. I have only one thought about that.

There is no better way to spend your money than on your health.

There is one more thing that I must caution you about if you hope to live a long and healthy life. It is simple: *Avoid drugs.* Prescription drugs can kill. The drug companies have a powerful hold on the medical treatment in this country and therefore a powerful affect on your health and longevity. It is my personal feeling that when you start on prescription drugs and take multiple drugs on an unlimited basis, you are in a death spiral taking you down to the graveyard. To give you an idea how huge and powerful the drug industry is, here are some facts:

The total expense for outpatient prescription drugs in this country in 2001 was 154.5 billion dollars. The cost of these drugs is spiraling up at a dramatic rate. Year 2001 showed a dramatic increase of 17% over the previous year continuing a well-established trend.

Let me remind you of something I said earlier. Most of these prescription drugs are a treatment, not a cure. All this money gives the drug companies their powerful influence on your medical doctors and your health.

When I was first married, in 1950, my first father-in-law gave me some excellent advice. I didn't know then how smart he was. He said, "Stay away from lawyers and doctors." I now repeat his advice to you. Stay away from lawyers and doctors when possible. Again, I want to be fair. If you break your arm or are seriously hurt in an accident, go to your MD at once. They are great and irreplaceable in certain areas.

In my opinion, the road to good health is not through toxins like drugs. One of two things will happen in the future. Either the medical doctors will become nutritionists or the nutritionists of today will become your doctors of tomorrow.

Longevity

While we are on the subject of living a long and healthy life, let me give you my current thinking on longevity. You might think I have really fallen off of my perch when you read this part, but please bear with me to the conclusion. I have always had a fear of dying and I wanted to avoid it as long as possible. I still do. Some years ago, I began to wonder how much influence our thinking has on our life expectancy. In other words, if we all think we're going to die in our 70's or 80's, does our thinking cause that to be true? We've already established that we should live well over 100 years.

There was an article some years ago about a man building dinosaurs in the Banning Pass. That's in between Palm Springs and Los Angeles, California. These dinosaurs are about 30' in height and made of a framework coated with concrete. According to this article, the man took two or three years to build each one. He had only finished one when the article was written. He planned to build about seven or eight in his lifetime. However, he was about 75 years old at that time. You can do the math as I did. I figured there's no way possible that he will ever finish all of them.

Years later, I finally figured it out. Oh, by the way, there are only two dinosaurs there now. I thought this guy must be nuts, but when you think about it, he was very bright. He lived his later years thinking that he would live much longer. Isn't that the attitude you want to have? Well, I don't know about you, but that's the attitude I want to have. In fact, here is my new attitude:

I sincerely believe that I will live to be 141 years old.

Now is when you're going to think my wife had better hide the bottle; I've surely had too much to drink. However, that is my attitude. I don't want to think I'm going to die tomorrow or next year or anytime soon. Whether or not I live that long is not the point. The point is my attitude of today. Do you get it now? Good!

It is great to have that attitude. I feel even better than I did before I developed this new attitude. So you see folks, at age 72 I'm only middle-aged now. Hope to see you around on my 141st birthday.

CHAPTER 15

MOTIVATION

I don't think one out of ten people with ALS will do what I've done to beat it. So, let me give you some motivation.

We've already discussed two of the problems 'pre-established beliefs' and 'habit.' I know we all have pre-established beliefs and habits that we don't want to change. However, when you are faced with an incurable disease like ALS, I don't understand why more of us are not motivated to do more. For that reason, I'm writing the following in an attempt to motivate you if you're one of those. Actually, I don't know why I should be so concerned about this because most people don't even do what their medical doctor tells them to do and I'm not even a MD.

OK, you have ALS or some other incurable neurological ailment. The way I see it, you have two choices:

1. Do nothing and die

   Or

2. Try

If you *don't try*, then you, by default, have selected alternative number one. **You're going to die.**

What's worse is this. Your quality of life will deteriorate to a nightmare.

Even if it means changing some of your pre-established beliefs or habits, don't you think it's worth it to try? I don't know how anyone can say no to that question. Perhaps you don't believe my story. Let me remind you that I am not *selling* anything. I share my experience freely with everyone. I have unquestionably stopped the progress of ALS *and* have steady improvement in all areas for seven years. Recognize also that I'm not the Lone Ranger. I have been in contact with seven other PALS who have shared my experience by following a program similar to mine.

There is every reason in the world to believe that I'm telling you the truth. There is no reason to not believe it. Additionally, there are books written by neurologists that agree with my ideas.

When I first put my program together, I knew I was right and I wanted to shout from the rooftops to all PALS in the world that I had the answer. I didn't do that because I wanted to prove to myself that my ideas were correct. I have now accomplished what I set out to do. So why do I not run to the rooftops and shout? The reason is too many people are skeptical and don't want to believe. Perhaps if I had MD behind my name more people would listen.

I am absolutely certain that toxins cause ALS. I'm absolutely certain that you will never beat ALS unless you remove the toxins from your body and avoid new toxins. Is that a hard fact to believe? It shouldn't be. It is pretty simple and straightforward. Let me repeat, I am also convinced that if you don't remove the toxins and avoid new ones, that you will die of ALS. You can extend your life a little bit with supplements. However, you can't really beat ALS unless you get to the *cause*. Toxins are the cause of ALS.

Remember the two choices I told you that you had earlier? Let's take choice number two and **TRY**.

CHAPTER 16

SUMMARY

In an attempt to make my story more interesting, I have jumped around a little bit. Let's do a skeletal review of my life with ALS in chronological order.

The ALS symptoms started in late 1990. I was first diagnosed in late '93. The progression of ALS was very slow at first, but remember I was taking a ton of supplements, including Vitamin E.

Following hip replacement surgery in July of '95, I began deteriorating faster. Additionally, I made the mistake of thinking my supplements were not helping me so I cut way back on them. I'm sure now that they were slowing my progression. However, I didn't appreciate that fact then.

In the fall of '96 we went to Loma Linda Medical Center for another opinion. This time they did *all* the invasive tests that were not done before. The tests came back negative for any other health problem. Diagnosis was again ALS; only this time it was for sure. I believe the trauma of the invasive tests contributed to a more rapid deterioration. There's a good side to this however. If things had not happened as they did, I probably would not be better today. The rapid deterioration is what sparked me into action. I finally decided to go all out! I had to give up my daily rations of coffee, beer and ice cream.

Within three months, I was on my way to recovery. By April of '97, I had overcome my choking problem and regained about 15 pounds.

I felt better and my overall strength was improving. My outlook on life had a 180 degree turnaround from the time of the November '96 diagnosis.

My improvement was slowed down some with the second hip replacement surgery in July '97.

In October '97, I joined the Sanofi Drug Trials. Sanofi was a drug company who was testing a new drug on ALS patients. I think it was supposed to rejuvenate or stimulate new growth in the nerves and brain cells. I thought this might be a great supplement to my program. However, there was no change in the rate of my improvement during the year I was on it. Additionally, there was no change when I started on Sanofi and there was no change after I stopped Sanofi.

"Well, it's July again, time for another surgery, right Eric?" Yep, sure enough. In July of '98, I had prostate surgery. Nothing too serious; just the usual roto-rooter service. Well, I survived the surgery with no ill effects. There was no affect on my ALS, probably because I took no pain pills or any other drug after the surgery.

It's now October 2000. There was no surgery in July 1999 or July 2000. Wow, what a relief! Oh no, I forgot, I had to have dental surgery in 1999, but it didn't happen until the first week of August. I had one root canal tooth. That is, a tooth where I had a root canal procedure done years ago. According to the book by Dr. Huggins, *"It's All in Your Head,"* a root canal tooth often times develops an infection at the base of the tooth. This infection can cause health problems. Apparently there is no way to know if you have an infection or not. Therefore, I decided that my root canal tooth had to go. Let me explain further. I said before if there is one chance in a thousand that something might adversely affect your ALS condition, then it should be eliminated. I finally decided that I couldn't afford not to have this tooth pulled.

Part of the procedure recommended by Dr. Huggins is the removal of the Periodontal Ligament that lies at the base of the tooth. I had to be referred to an oral surgeon for this procedure. I heard the doctor say as he removed the ligament that there was no sign of infection. I'm still happy I did it because I don't have to worry now about whether or not there is an infection.

Let me tell you about an interesting side note here. The surgery was done with local anesthetic only. No pain pills. I did take a Valium an hour beforehand to lessen my anxiety. About two hours after arriving home, the local anesthetic had worn off and I had a fair amount of pain. I had just read a very interesting book on the use of magnets for pain and for speeding up the healing process. The name of the book is *"Healing with Magnets"* by Gary Null, Ph.D. I decided to try out the magnet idea and to test my own PMA. Glenna helped me by wrapping a magnet in a scarf and tying the scarf around my head with the magnet directly over the area of pain. I then repeated to myself over and over for about twenty minutes the following: "I don't want any pain. Pain; go away. I don't need any pain, etc., etc." I'm serious when I say twenty minutes. I watched the clock. After about thirty minutes, the pain reduced to about half what it was. In one hour, it was completely gone. I then removed the magnet. I know this doesn't prove anything. The pain might have gone away on its own. Remember however, I took no pain pills; not even an aspirin. I had absolutely no pain for about five days. Then, the pain returned but only at about half the severity. It lasted for about three more days and then the pain ended. I know this doesn't prove that magnets are a cure-all or that they have any effect at all. However, in my opinion, this experience supports what Dr. Null said in his book. Magnets are a great supplement to the healing process.

There is one other thing that occurred during this time period that I should mention. Around November of '98, I got real tired of my diet and thought it was about time to add some foods which I sorely missed – ice cream and milk. I really missed ice cream! I ate ice cream for about six months until May of '99. Toward the end of that six-month period, I realized my improvement had ceased and I was having BM accidents again and frequently. In a talk with my nutritionist, I admitted my ice cream habit. She told me to cut it out. I explained to her that I had been drinking milk and eating ice cream for decades before ALS with no problem. She suggested that two years without ice cream and milk that my body had ceased to make the necessary enzymes to digest milk. Of course, I had to agree and went back on my diet. That immediately solved the diarrhea problem. Also, within almost no time, I noticed mild improvement again. In looking back, I think now that the milk I was drinking and the milk in the ice cream was causing diarrhea. I think the sugar in the ice cream was slowing down my improvement.

We are approaching the end of 2001 so it's been almost five years since I started my program. My rate of improvement seems to have picked up just lately, particularly since I started with my new 'alternative treatment' M.D. My improvement is noticeable in my stepping in and out of the shower, getting up out of bed, and getting in and out of the truck. I seem to be getting a little stronger and more flexible. It would appear that I'm another year or two away from reaching my current goal of walking and talking comfortably.

It has been eleven years since my first diagnosis and fourteen years since my first symptoms. I would like to encourage you to follow a program similar to mine and here's why. There are many others who have survived ALS for ten years or more. I am not the Lone Ranger. Let me tell you about a few whom I have had direct contact with by e-mail. I don't know their entire history, but I'll tell you the little bit that I do know. Here they are:

1. Heavy supplement program including Vitamin E and Grape Seed Extract. Number of amalgams unknown.
2. Supplement and diet program similar to mine. Number of amalgams unknown.
3. Supplement and diet program similar to mine. All amalgams removed.
4. Supplement program. All amalgams removed plus removal of one root canal tooth and Periodontal Ligament.
5. Supplement program. Never had any amalgams. He is a retired dentist and has only gold fillings.
6. Strict diet and massive supplements. Still has two or three amalgams.

If you include me, I make number seven. I'm on a strict diet and massive supplements. I only had two amalgams and they were removed.

All these people are long-term survivors of ALS of nine years or more and without any breathing apparatus or peg tube inserted directly into the stomach for feeding. That's pretty remarkable. Make note of the fact that everyone of them is on some kind of a diet and supplement program. Also, most of them have no amalgam fillings. A common thread with all of them is that they are all following the same general idea. That is detox, diet and supplements.

Update – June 2001

I have just recently been in contact by e-mail with another PALS who has enjoyed steady improvement for two years so he makes number eight (including me). Here is what is very interesting about him. He is following a program very close to my own and that just tickles me pink. Why? Because it would seem to give my program even more credibility. He is following every aspect:

1. **PMA** – You must believe
2. **Prayer** – Don't overlook this one
3. **Colonic hydrotherapy** – very important detox procedure
4. **Removal of amalgams** – a source of mercury poisoning
5. **Diet** – to avoid toxins *and* properly nourish the body
6. **Supplements** – help the body heal itself
7. **Chelation** – number one detox procedure

Before we part company, I have a few more thoughts on attitude that I would like to share with you.

My first father-in-law (I'm now on number three) told me one time "Don't ever expect anything and you will never be disappointed."

The formula for DISAPPOINTMENT is where *expectation exceeds reality.* The formula for HAPPINESS is where *reality exceeds expectation.*

"Well, that's fine and dandy, Eric, but doesn't that conflict with your statements about Positive Mental Attitude?" Yes and no; it is a matter of selection. You will see what I mean in a minute.

Have you ever heard of the Serenity Prayer? Even if you have, I'm going to repeat it here so we can discuss it. I think this is one of the greatest pieces of writing ever put to the pen.

"GOD GRANT ME THE SERENITY
TO ACCEPT THE THINGS
I CANNOT CHANGE,
THE COURAGE TO CHANGE
THE THINGS I CAN,
AND THE WISDOM TO KNOW
THE DIFFERENCE."

This is truly a classic statement. How many people do you know who go around complaining and worrying about things they can't change? For example, they complain about things over which they have no control like the weather or not enough hours in the day. What a waste of time and energy that is. They would be so much better off channeling their thoughts and efforts into another area as the second part of the prayer states. If you don't like something the way it is and you are in a position to affect it, then by all means you should attempt to change it.

Here is the real meat of the prayer. "The *wisdom* to know the difference." Is that beautiful or what? You see, there is the real problem with many of us. We fail to recognize the difference between what we can change and what we can't change. Therefore, your selection of the two choices in expectation, as we discussed above, is based on whether or not you can change something. Example: You can't change the weather. I hope you have the wisdom to know that. Therefore, do not expect everyday to be sunny and you will not be disappointed. Get the idea? I'm sure you do. Following the message of the Serenity Prayer could go a long way toward making anyone a happier, more pleasant person. The bottom line is don't attempt to change something that you can't. However, you should attempt to change whatever you can. Recognize that you can change the outcome of ALS. This is where the wisdom part comes in; where *you* have to make the *selection*. The majority of MD's will tell you that ALS is terminal and incurable. I'm attempting to convince you that they are wrong. You can beat ALS. I have done it and I'm not the only one. Don't give up. Use your *wisdom* and *select* the path of *change.*

Part of the problem here is that human frailty I mentioned earlier. That is, one's ability to ignore hard evidence when it conflicts with pre-established beliefs. "Don't confuse me with the facts; my mind is already made up." Don't let this happen to you. You must believe that *you* can beat ALS.

The critics can say what they want, but I know my program, at the very least, has already extended my life. My improvement simply cannot be coincidental. No other PALS that I know of has ever improved from ALS by *accident.* The improvement always coincides with some specific program that they have followed.

I am really certain that I have overcome ALS and I will probably live another 20 years or more (unless I'm hit by a truck).

When I was on the Sanofi Drug Trials, the doctor at Scripps would examine me every month. After seeing my improvement, month after month, he finally remarked one day. "Eric, you will have to get something else to kill you, because ALS isn't going to do it."

UPDATES TO THE BOOK "ERIC IS WINNING"

The following Updates were written after the book was originally published.
They are included for your information.

November 2004

Although I have improved slightly in the last two or three years, my improvement has been very slow. I just discovered why. My latest hair analysis indicates that my mercury level had gone back up a lot. The only explanation that is possible, is that I have been eating some fish in the last couple of years. I now believe that you cannot eat any fish no matter what kind or where they are caught.

Irritable Bowel Syndrome (IBS) is another illness for which the doctors do not have any cure. My doctor suggested a prescription drug for my IBS but after I read about it, I decided it was too risky for a PALS. The doctors say they don't know what causes IBS. Well, duh! There can only be one explanation. It must be something you ate. I did the same thing that I did with ALS. I gathered a lot of information and went on an extreme diet and I have now cured my IBS. However, during that time, I was not improving my ALS condition at all. After eliminating the IBS problem, I then returned to treating my ALS condition. I had to do more chelation with DMPS and more chelation with LL's Magnetic Clay baths and now my mercury level is way down again.

Now, for the really interesting part. I'm really not what you would call a religious person. However, I do believe in God and I do believe in prayer. About a year ago, I changed my prayer from something like "God, help me find a way to beat this ALS" to something like this "God, I think I have suffered long enough with my ALS. Could you now help me speed up my recovery?" Well, what do you know? It certainly appears as though He has answered my prayers. I have learned about more new treatments for ALS in the last year than in all the thirteen years before that. The latest treatment that I have discovered is in the form of a supplement. Now, I have to be very careful to not oversell this one, BUT I am so convinced about the benefits that it's hard to control my enthusiasm. Here's why I say that. Every movement I make with my arms, legs, etc. is limited. When I make a move that is the best I have done recently, I grade that a "10." If I make a move that goes beyond my previous limit, I call that an "11." I have had a great many "11's" recently and I have been taking the supplement for three months now. Additionally, I have not had any setbacks. The improvement seems to be more consistent. The possible explanation for this is that this supplement improves the immune system. The supplement is glyconutrients.

Glenna and I just returned from a three-day stay at a gambling casino in Laughlin, Nevada. During the three days, I decided to put this idea to a test. I threw all caution to the wind and ate anything I wanted including a double scoop of ice cream every night, a cinnamon roll in the morning with my latte, and much more. I not only did not have any setbacks, but I feel like I actually improved during that time.

I must admit that I'm doing several more things than just taking the new supplement. I've done more chelation and clay baths. I've done Human Growth Hormone well over a year, etc. However, the only thing new has been the supplement and coincidental with that I've had many "11's."

Glyconutrients

These glyconutrients were only discovered about ten years ago. Even though there have been many articles written and published in magazines and medical journals, they are not well known.

It is my understanding that glyconutrients only occur in fruits and vegetables and then they only occur within the last few days of the ripening process. Most foods are harvested when they are a little green, and they do not contain the glyconutrients. Therefore, most of the nutrients are not in the average person's food supply. Even if you buy organically grown fruit and veggies, they were probably picked prior to when they were fully ripened. Have you ever eaten fresh fruit such as a peach that you just picked from the tree? If so, you're familiar with the vastly better taste than what you buy in the market. This tells me that something really does occur in the last few days of the ripening process. These nutrients are said to be ESSENTIAL for good health just like air and water is essential for life. Further, these nutrients are essential for cell communication with one and another. Without communication, our immune system simply won't work.

If you've read my book, you know that I believe that toxins are the cause of ALS and many other illnesses. I just know that I'm right about that, **but** I now must admit that if our immune system was working properly, then the toxins might not be harmful to us. That may explain why only some of us get ALS, for example, and others do not, even though we may have many of the same toxins in our bodies.

It appears to me that there is a correlation between my improvement and my pH level being more alkaline. For example, all during my IBS diet, I had absolutely no improvement at all and I was on a more acidic diet to cure the IBS. Since then, I've been taking the new supplement and I've been on a more alkaline diet and I now have more improvement. Even prior to my IBS diet, I could never maintain a pH of 7.0 consistently. It would be up one day and down the next. Since I'm on the new supplement, my pH level is consistently 6.8 to 7.2. It appears to me that the glyconutrients have finally enabled me to correct my pH problem.

The above theory about glyconutrients and my own personal experience of the last few months have convinced me that these nutrients really **are essential**. Based on this, I have created a new list of the absolute minimum essential items that I would do. You will find a list of minimum items at the end of Phase One in the Regimen Outline.

Now I have a new prayer. My new prayer goes like this:

> "Thank you God for all that I have and all that you've done to help me with ALS."

I feel like all my prayers have been answered and I'm now writing the last chapter in my ALS experience and it's all positive.

January 2005

My eyesight just improved. Before I tell you more about this recent improvement, let me lay some groundwork. I had a desk job most of my life and about thirty years ago I wore glasses to read anything and everything. One day I was reading and the words were blurring. I took off my glasses and the words were clear. I could then read normal print without my glasses. I threw my glasses away. This had to be the result of adding a new supplement to my diet. I added Vitamin B Complex to my normal multi-vitamin.

Now for more on my recent vision improvement. I clearly have 20/20 eyesight but for about eight years now I've been reading the stock market quotes with reading glasses. As you know, that is extremely fine print. Well, the other day I read the stock market quotes without my glasses and very clearly. So, again, I've had remarkable improvement in my eyesight. The only recent change has been adding glyconutrients and that must be the reason for the improvement.

However, there is a forerunner to this event and may have something to do with the change also. I just recently received the results of my fourth hair analysis. My second hair analysis indicated lower heavy metals than my first hair analysis. The third hair analysis showed higher heavy metals than the second hair analysis.

I'm sure this was due to my eating fish again. In addition to eliminating all fish from my diet, I have had seventeen foot baths with LL's Magnetic Clay during the last several months. Now, here is the kicker. My fourth recent hair analysis showed my heavy metals to be way lower than any previous hair analysis. Every single heavy metal is down way below the acceptable minimum. My Dr. Rouzier said he had never seen one so low.

I receive a lot of e-mail wanting to know how I'm doing currently. Although I've had a great deal of improvement since my clay foot baths and my discovery of glyconutrients, I'm still not 100% recovered. I'm able to move my feet around much better recently making it much easier to transfer. I can step forward with my right foot better than ever but of course only with a walker. The only remaining problems are walking and talking and finger dexterity. My foot movement and my finger dexterity has improved a lot in the last two months.

My speech is greatly improved and I'm dictating this to Glenna. There are times when I can speak quite normally.

You might be interested to know that I receive e-mail from many people who are following my regimen and are enjoying improvement.

You might also be interested in my reply to those people who don't have improvement and I hear from them too. Often times they tell me that they have followed my program but have no improvement. However, after some discussion I learn that they haven't. That's one of the reasons why I developed my Regimen Outline. If you're not having improvement, the first thing you should do is review my Regimen Outline.

If you have done everything and still have no improvement, then here is my standard response.

Remember, toxins cause ALS and probably all other neuro-degenerative illnesses. Therefore, you either have not done enough detox and/or you have not eliminated one or more toxins in your environment.

There is no magic formula, single treatment or supplement that will beat ALS. Please believe this. You must do more. If you approach your problem with PMA and continue a variety of Phase One treatments, I know you will eventually succeed.

Glenna and I wish you well.

Bye for now.

February 2005

Here is some information on avoiding toxins that could save your life if you're suffering from any neuro-degenerative illness. In the book, I devoted one full chapter to avoiding toxins. However, I did not include this information which is fairly new to me.

More and more frequently we hear from PALS who are enjoying improvement. Now and then, we hear from someone who is not. My thinking is refined now and then by what I learn. It is my thought that if you have followed all of the suggested treatments and have no improvement, or have rapidly progressing symptoms, then you may have a major toxin in your environment which you may not be aware of.

Here are three true stories illustrating what I mean.

LEAD

A married couple returned home from a trip to Europe. Shortly, they both began to develop symptoms of a neuro-degenerative illness. The doctors had no clue about the cause. Then, they sold their home and moved, and soon their symptoms were improving. After two or three weeks, their symptoms reappeared. To make a long story short, they finally traced it to two coffee cups they bought in Europe and began using everyday. Then, the cups were packed away when they moved. When they began using the cups again, their symptoms reappeared. They had the coffee cups tested and they were leeching lead. Lead is toxic.

FUNGUS & WATER POLLUTION

Erin Brokovich was the heroine in Hinckley, California where she discovered that hundreds of people in the area were suffering various health problems because their water supply was polluted by a nearby chemical plant. Please note that the local doctors who were treating all these people did not have a clue about the cause. Meanwhile Erin, with no medical background, figured it out. Wow! Sometime after that, Erin began to have symptoms similar to ALS. The problem was traced to fungus in the walls of her home that was inside the walls and not visible. If you've ever had any water leak in your home or in your automobile, you could have fungus in there. Fungus creates toxic spores that travel through the air and infect the human body.

WOOD FLOORING PRESERVATIVE

I read a magazine article about a couple who bought a home and had new wooden flooring installed. Soon after moving in the man developed ALS-like symptoms. They traced it to the flooring and they moved out. The symptoms immediately went away. Apparently wood used for flooring must have a preservative. The preservative they are currently using is highly toxic. This preservative can create a vapor for a long, long time after installation. Environmentalists tried to have it banned but politics got in the way and it is still being used another few years. In the meantime, many people will die.

I recently lost a friend to ALS. In looking back on the situation, I now believe I know the cause. Here are the clues. He and his wife moved into a new home that had hardwood floors throughout the home. Immediately after moving in, his symptoms of ALS began. He deteriorated rapidly but even more so after he quit work and was confined to the home 24 hours a day. His hair analysis indicated very low heavy metals. Although he and his wife followed many suggestions in my outline, he was dead in less than one year. That's why I believe when progression is that rapid, then there must be a major toxin in the environment, and in this case, it could well have been the wood flooring preservative.

Well, that's the end of the three stories, but they should provide you with some ideas about what you may be up against. No one can know your environment better than you. Therefore, you must be the detective.

March 2005

You will find at the end of Phase One of the latest Regimen Outline, a heading **Conclusion of Phase One**. The items listed I believe are absolutely essential for anyone's good health. One of them is the pH factor. I'm writing about this now because I believe most people grossly under estimate this. Additionally, these items are inter-related. You must correct your pH to alkaline. Detox, glyconutrients, avoiding all toxins and diet are all part of correcting your pH. Based on my latest experience you may want to add Terramin clay to your diet. It is now my belief that the main reason you are acidic and are sick is because you are mineral deficient. Terramin clay includes many minerals in their natural form.

I first read about the pH factor when I bought some coral calcium. Coral calcium alone did not correct my pH. Then I began taking Glyconutrients several months ago and my pH improved. I thought it was OK but I was not checking it everyday.

About three weeks ago I decided that it was time for me to exercise my legs more. In the supermarket parking lot they have a pipe enclosure about ten feet long for market baskets. It was just right for my walking exercise. I walked up and back for one lap and a total of twenty feet. The first day I did only one lap. The second day I did two laps. The third day I did three laps. Then it rained for a couple of days and I walked six laps. It rained again and after a couple of days I returned to walking but could only do two laps and it was more difficult than doing six. I knew something had changed but I did not know what. The next evening I was doing knee bends and it was difficult. I knew something was wrong and it finally occurred to me to check my pH. I checked it and I was very acidic with a reading of 6.0. I had recently received a jar of Terramin which is a clay to be used internally. The label says "Rich in calcium and trace minerals" among other things. When your system is acidic, they say you are mineral deficient, so this seemed like a good thing to try. I took one teaspoonful in a full glass of water once a day in the morning on an empty stomach. Three days later I returned to the supermarket parking lot and I walked **eight** laps with ease. I came home and immediately checked my pH and it was 7.4. What an amazing experience.

I found that I had to increase my Terramin clay to one teaspoon twice a day to have greater consistency of my pH. I find it necessary to check my pH two or three times a day to be sure that it is where I want it and it is now.

You can order Terramin clay from the following:

Maryanne Maldonado
e-mail *namaste9@comcast.net*
phone 520 219-2379

Several times in the last few months I have experienced this coincidence of weakness and low pH. However, this recent walking experience is the most dramatic ever.

Perhaps you can now see why I believe so much in the need to correct your pH. I now believe that you'll never get better unless you do this **and** the other items in the conclusion of Phase One.

DR. AKIN & HAIR ANALYSIS

Here is some really great news. I've just learned about another source for a hair analysis. A Dr. Akin in Ohio uses a different laboratory and they provide a more elaborate hair analysis. You will find more information about Dr. Akin in my latest Regimen Outline. I am truly impressed with her and this new source of hair analysis.

April 2005

STEM CELL AND CHINA

Before you cash in your piggy bank and spend $25,000 to $50,000 to go to China for the stem cell surgery, you may want to rethink that. I was ready to go there myself when I received the first report from someone who had been there. The initial report sounded perfect with 100% success rate, etc. However, the latest of two reports I have received indicate problems. Many patients have recurring symptoms and a few may have died.

Here is my opinion for what it's worth:

> Any treatment that does not address the cause of ALS is doomed to eventual failure, even though it may provide temporary improvement.

The cause of ALS is toxins.

You must first detoxify your body and eliminate every toxin in your environment before you can expect permanent improvement.

I have long said that treating ALS requires different treatments in Phase One from Phase Two.

The PURPOSE of Phase One is to eliminate the CAUSE of ALS. Then you can move into Phase Two and the purpose is restoring your body. I feel it is critical that you understand that treatments to detoxify are Phase One treatments and treatments to restore the body are Phase Two treatments.

For well over a year now, I have said repeatedly that stem cell treatments may be great. However, stem cell replacement is clearly a Phase Two treatment because it does not treat the CAUSE. This recent experience in China seems to prove my theory.

Now, if you've done all the Phase One treatments already, and then go to China, that may be OK. A friend of mine went there and had good results because he had done Phase One before going to China. However, I am not recommending the China solution.

You may not have to go to China. I am experimenting right now with a stem cell treatment available locally without surgery. I'll let you know more when I know more in a later update. See the Regimen Outline.

UPDATE ON MY CONDITION

Did you ever see a fat man with ALS? Probably not because by the time you are diagnosed with ALS you've already lost a lot of weight and no amount of food intake will change that. I weighed 155 before ALS. My lowest weight since was 136. Then, the last couple of years I've been right around 143 and never anymore than that. I had not weighed myself in several months until the other day.

I NOW WEIGH 149.

So if you want to see a fat man with ALS just stick around. 149 is the most I have weighed in over eight years. I don't believe any PALS ever gains weight unless they have already beaten the illness as I have. I believe I owe the newly gained weight to the following:

1. I have balanced my pH to the alkaline side.
2. By my latest hair analysis, my heavy metals are nearly zero.
3. I believe I have eliminated every possible toxin from my environment including my home, my colon, my teeth and gums, etc.
4. Glyconutrients.

I urge you to review the latest revision of my Regimen Outline found here on this same web site. It probably has more information than the previous outline in your book.

Here's to your health,

Fat Eric

May 2005

GOOD NEWS

You might be interested to know that other PALS are following some of my suggestions and HAVING IMPROVEMENT. Now and then I receive an e-mail telling me about someone's success. Here are excerpts from a John McInnes e-mail of 4-24-05 that is particularly interesting.

"Dear Eric, you'll never guess what, I'm back from London having had the root canal tooth removed along with the periodontal liga- ment and the socket cleaned out with a dental burr in order for the bone to heal properly–all in accordance with Hal Huggins and I have a dramatic improvement in my symptoms! It's unbelievable– my voice is so much better, my swallowing and walking are both much improved, I can hardly believe it. I still have to remove 4 nickel based crowns and am returning in 2 weeks to get this done. Thank you Eric for telling me about Hal Huggins, I am so grateful. I do think that if I had a mouthful of mercury amalgams with ALS I would follow Huggins protocol to the letter and remove them in absolute sequence as he says that for ALS and Leukemia this has given improvements and the quadrant method hasn't and let's face it he is the expert–please consider mentioning this in your book."

"I still have a long way to go but now I believe that anything is possible–it has been a great boost for morale."

"I'm still doing the clay baths and now that I have "Wellness Water" arriving direct to my bath I find the clay dissolves so much more easily and I have more dark residue left in the bath."

"Love to you and Glenna, Jehan McInnes.

Best regards,

John McInnes"

The above e-mail from John McInnes should be a reminder to all of you that you must do everything the right way. If you try to cut corners, you probably will not get the results you expect. All of you should review the latest revision of the Regimen Outline and make sure you are doing all the right things and in the right order.

Looking forward to your improvement and receiving more e-mail like the one John McInnes just sent me.

We wish you well.

June 2005

ELECTROLYTES

It simply continues to amaze me. Since I changed my prayer over a year ago, more new information about treatments for ALS keeps coming my way. Here's another one.

Three different PALS wrote to me about a Dr. Patricia Kane at the Haverford Wellness Center who is having success treating ALS patients. I contacted her and I will be starting on her treatment protocol soon. However, she first told me about electrolytes and I started on a product called E-Lyte that she recommended. Almost immediately I had improvement in my overall strength. If I were you, I would add E-Lyte to my regimen at once.

If any of you are interested in more information about Dr. Kane's protocol, you may contact her office:

Haverford Wellness Center
Dr. Domenick Braccia
Dr. Patricia Kane
2010 West Chester Pike
Suite 310
Havertown, PA 19083
Phone: 610 924-0600
Fax: 610 924-0600 *www.haverfordwellness.com*

NOTE:

I'm currently taking four capfuls of E-Lyte in a glass of pure water four times a day.

Coincidentally I just received an e-mail from another PALS whose ALS condition is improving. He believes that a primary cause of ALS is dehydration; in other words, you're not drinking enough water. I only try treatments that are logical and make sense. Obviously drinking more water is well-recognized as necessary for good health, but it may be far more important than any of us realize. In addition to the water, you need electrolytes.

The "L.A. Times" recently had an article about water in the Health Section of their paper. According to this article, too much water can kill you. Now that sounds nutty, doesn't it? Here's the explanation. If you are heavy into sports activities and drink a lot of pure water, you may be flushing out all the electrolytes in your system and that is bad. The complete statement is that too much water WITHOUT ELECTROLYTES may be hazardous to your health. I don't know about you, but I am planning to continue my E-Lyte and increase my dose of it in the future and drink more and more water. Drinking water is a requisite for removing toxins from your body. Additionally, in order for your cells to function correctly, you must have adequate hydration.

VITAMIN B-1

I will tell you more about this in next month's update, but I cannot resist telling you now about Vitamin B-1. Based on what I've recently learned and what I already knew, I have increased my daily intake of Vitamin B-1 to 400 mg a day. Vitamin B-1 injections are far superior to taking B-1 orally. I'm currently taking 200 mg by injection daily plus 200 more orally. I'll tell you much more about this in next month's update but I think it works.

MANNATECH

The June 6th issue of Business Week's cover story is the Top 100 Small Companies, Mannatech is listed at #6!!! I buy some of their vitamins including Ambrotose. I believe they have high-quality products and apparently a lot of other people do too. Just thought you might want to know this.

July 2005

pH FACTOR

Balancing your pH to a more alkaline level is difficult; at least it has been for me. It has taken me several months. Assuming others of you may have the same problem, here are my thoughts based on my personal experience.

I don't believe there is any one supplement that will correct your pH. If you find one that seems to, I question whether or not it is really doing the job right. Also, I don't believe that you can correct your pH by diet alone. However, diet is important. It seems to me that it is more important to add alkaline foods to your diet than it is to eliminate acidic foods. I eat eggs in the morning three out of four days and I eat meat four out of five days. However, I drink one 16 oz. Starbucks Chai tea latte with SOY MILK everyday. Soy milk and soy lecithin are alkaline. Of course my diet still includes a lot of fresh veggies and no white potatoes, white rice, or pasta.

Here is a list of all the items I am now taking, each of which I believe has contributed to the correction of my pH:

> Ambrotose – 4 tsp. added to my yogurt twice a day
> Terramin Clay – 1 tsp. added to 8 oz. water twice a day
> Multi-Vitamin – containing 500 mg of calcium daily
> Weekly IV of vitamins/minerals
> Electrolytes (brand name E-Lyte) – 4 capfuls in 12 oz. water four times a day
> Chai Tea Latte with soy milk

This is not everything I take daily but only those items that I think have a direct bearing on my pH. When your system is acidic, you are also mineral deficient usually. I think adding minerals may be the main thing to do. The Terramin Clay, E-Lyte, the Multi-vitamin and the IV all contain minerals.

Each of these items when added to my regimen improved my pH. However, my pH was never consistent until now. Currently, I check my pH once or twice a day and I normally have a reading of 7.2 or higher. Even after all this, I still have the occasional day when my pH is below 7.0. However, that is now very rare. I cannot explain that occasional drop in pH, but again it is rare.

Regardless of what your health problem may be (cancer, ALS, heart, etc.), correcting your pH may be the most important thing you can do other than detoxify.

The pH factor is probably the best kept health care secret of all time.

According to what I have read, medical school does not teach nutrition. Therefore, most MD's don't know about pH and its importance. However, I believe balancing your pH to more alkaline is absolutely critical to your improvement.

GLYCONUTRIENTS

On February 19, 2003, a remarkable article in The Journal of the American Medical Association (JAMA) on research from Johns Hopkins Medical School reported for the first time that donor stem cells crossed the blood brain barrier and became neurons in the recipient's brain. This is an important finding because neurons are the most highly advanced functional cells in the body; they control all brain and muscle functions. This is a recent revolutionary discovery about the potential to repair and regenerate the human brain.

Early research on glyconutrients (the necessary sugars) suggests that by adding glyconutrients to the human diet, there is an increase in production of one's bone marrow stem cells.

Until the JAMA article, Dr. McDaniel's science team had not been able to explain how adults with Alzheimer's, Parkinson's, and Huntington's and children with cerebral palsy, leukodystrophy, Down syndrome, autism and FAS {fetal alcohol syndrome} experience restorations in brain function with the addition of glyconutrients and other micronutrients to their diet.

Prior to this knowledge in 2003 from JAMA, there was no reasonable scientific explanation of how the many individuals with presumed permanent brain injury from strokes, trauma or neuro-degenerative disorders could heal and regain lost central nervous system function that physicians and scientists had regarded as permanent and irreversible.

Our new understanding of glyconutrients stimulating the development of one's bone marrow stem cells, which have the capacity to develop into any cell the body needs, provides us with a scientific understanding of how such unparalleled restorations of brain function can be induced by dietary supplementation of glyconutrients.

IMPROVEMENT LETTER FROM BRENDA & JAMES

"Eric Is Winning"

I just wanted to tell you that your book is outstanding. My husband was just diagnosed with ALS in March. He wasn't even able to walk. Now he walks with no problems. I'm following your book strictly, it is improving his health.

I just wanted to say " THANK YOU" for taking the time to write this book. It's helped our family tremendously.

God Bless You,

Brenda & James Lisinski

Ashley, Nathan, Jamee

August 2005

TOXINS CAUSE ALS AND MUCH MORE

It is my absolute belief that toxins cause ALS and all of the forty or more other neuro-degenerative illnesses such as Alzheimer's, MS, Parkinson's, etc. It is also my belief that once you have any of these neuro illnesses that your immune system has been all but destroyed. Therefore, it is IMPERATIVE that you not only detoxify your body but eliminate every toxin in your body, in your environment, and in your diet. Overlooking any one of these could be fatal. One such toxin that is often overlooked is mycoplasma. Mycoplasma are little bugs that successfully hide in other cells in your colon and are difficult to detect. Here is an e-mail from another PALS who has tested positive for Mycoplasma and included is some valuable information:

*   *   *

"Thank you, Eric, for your comments and understanding. Please find below the results of my Mycoplasma blood test. My regimen outline will follow in a separate e-mail.

My blood samples were forwarded to Medical Diagnostic Laboratories, 2439 Kuser Road, Hamilton, NJ 08690-3303, Telephone 609-570-1000; fax: 609-570-1050; E-mail: *www.mdlab.com*. **The results were positive for Mycoplasma fermentans.** The only known source for me would have been vaccinations I received.

The nice part about this find is everything you've done and expressed in your book and updates, is exactly the treatment that should be followed (drug free), especially glyconutrients with the strong support offered to the glial cells and its correlation in the eventual destruction of the bacteria. The 8 glyconutrients needed by the cells are not readily available in our foods today; some are but not all. I feel good and your regimen has given me great hope.

Thank you again,
Joe Martin
jjm@pei.sympatico.ca
Prince Edward Island, Canada"

*   *   *

Joe Martin also sent me his entire supplement list as recommended. I believe the most significant supplements are as follows:

Glyconutrients

Two natural antibiotics; colloidal silver and olive leaf extract.

May I urge you to not overlook the possibility that you may have Mycoplasma in your colon?

The main reason Glyconutrients are included is because they are ESSENTIAL for your immune system to function properly and they are not normally in our diets.

Glenna and I receive a lot of e-mail from a lot of PALS with many questions. They rarely include questions about pH or Glyconutrients. This leads me to believe that many of you may be overlooking these two items. I wish to emphasize the following statement and I believe my word choices are better than bold print. I hope I don't offend anyone with my bold words, but I must say this.

If you are not maintaining an alkaline balance in your pH AND taking a therapeutic dose of Glyconutrients, you are a fool or you have holes in your head. Again I hope this does not offend; I am your friend and I only say this for emphasis.

You may also want to review the Regimen Outline to make sure that you're doing all you can to beat ALS.

The reason I am so emphatic today is because I've watched two friends with ALS die recently. I know for a fact that they did not do everything in my Regimen Outline. It is hard to stand by and watch when you know that they are not helping themselves.

Here's to you and your health; you know what to do, now do it! Glenna and I wish you well.

September 2005

Sorry to be late with this update, but something exciting delayed me. Last Saturday friends of ours, Jake and Becky, met us at Starbucks and told us about their previous two weeks at a Holistic detox center in San Diego, California. Glenna and I were so excited about it that we called immediately and found they had a cancellation and we booked a one week stay starting the next day Sunday. Our stay at the clinic was full of events that we will never forget. They provide three meals a day of raw food, some of which is grown right there on their premises organically. How good can it get. They provide a schedule of great classes; very educational about health. I went there with the "dream" of riding in on my scooter and "walking" out. But my real "hope" was that I would see some recognizable change. I was not disappointed. We arrived Sunday at 3:00 PM. By Monday evening I was tired. However, Tuesday morning I thought that I could lift my feet slightly higher making it easier to move my feet around when transferring. Wednesday morning it seemed the improvement was a little more. Then Thursday morning the inevitable happened. I had bowel problems. It is really amazing that I was able to last that long. That caused us to terminate our stay and travel home.

I'm purposely leaving out the details of their regimen because you just have to go there. However, you can only go there if you're independent or with a caregiver. They do not have handicap rooms, so you must be able to handle that. I did not lose any weight during the week, but you might, so a word of caution. Glenna, however, lost seven pounds in four days. By the way, there is no radio, TV, or newspapers and they don't allow perfume, hair spray, aftershave lotion, or any other "smelly stuff" on your skin.

Now I was taking several supplements before I went there and I left them ALL home.

I believe my slight improvement proves one of my theories and that is you must do many different TYPES of detox. I don't want to sound like I'm selling you on this; I just want you to know about it so I won't tell you anymore. If you want more info, you can call them. Here is their phone number:

Optimum Health Institute
Phone (619) 464-3346 or (800) 993-4325
Web site: *www.optimumhealth.org*

Eric

October 2005

MORE ABOUT MY SAN DIEGO EXPERIENCE
(See September Update)

After my San Diego experience, I have been analyzing what's happening and why. Here are my thoughts. First of all, let me remind you that in my book I discuss that I've done three things that no doubt are responsible for my last nine years of improvement. Generally speaking, I felt that I had to:

1. Eliminate toxins in my environment.
2. Eliminate toxins in my diet
3. Detoxify my body

Even though I knew this, I never fully got into organic food for my diet. That may explain why I have been so slow in recovering.

Now this is important. The only explanation for my dramatic improvement in San Diego is that they serve only RAW, UNCOOKED and ORGANIC food, water, and drinks. I am now thoroughly convinced that one must eat strictly ORGANIC food and as much as reasonable raw food. What I really mean is 100% organic, not 75% or even 90%. If you cannot find organic food in your neighborhood, then you had better move. There is simply no acceptable excuse because your life may depend upon it.

When we left San Diego, we were so hungry for regular food that we stopped at a restaurant. I had two eggs and two pancakes. This caused me a major setback immediately. Glenna had to lift my feet to help me get in our truck. How discouraging.

I am now on 99% organic food. Fortunately, a new Clark's Nutrition market opened up near us that is 90% all organic food. I now eat two or three organic eggs cooked in organic butter. I have one piece of organic toast with organic butter. I eat a homemade salad of raw organic veggies with a homemade organic buttermilk dressing. I follow that with steamed organic veggies and organic steak (beef or lamb).

I have fully recovered from my setback from the eggs and pancakes and am now better than I was when I left San Diego. This can only be the result of all organic food in my diet and other things I've been doing the last few months.

Here is what I've been doing. Remember, I've already been through "mucho" detox and I'm now in Phase Two (restoration).

1. 200 mg of B-1 injections daily AND 200 mg of B-1 orally
2. Dr. Kane's Lipid IV twice a week
3. Electrolytes – 2 capfuls of E-Lyte in each of four 12 oz. glasses of water daily (two before breakfast and two before dinner)
4. Glyconutrients – 4 TEASPOONS Ambrotose twice a day in organic yogurt. Note: It has been proven that Glyconutrients cause the body to produce more of its own stem cells.
5. A daily dose of live cells orally. See live cell therapy in Phase Two of the Regimen Outline revision 12/05.
6. Two capsules daily of Sea Vegg – can be ordered at 1-800-672-9118 or see web site www.tryseavegg.com
7. About every two to three weeks I have a vitamin/mineral/glutathione IV by Dr. Rouzier.
8. I have eliminated all other supplements and I have eliminated Human Growth Hormone and Colostrum.
9. We have eliminated cooking eggs in a teflon coated pan. Teflon is toxic.
10. One 16. oz. Chai Tea Latte with soy milk at Starbucks daily.

I believe everything I'm doing now is effective and is helping me. I'm very satisfied with my improvement in the last two weeks. I have had more improvement in the last few weeks than any other similar time period in eight years.

You might be interested to know that my fifth and most recent hair analysis by Dr. Akin indicates a lower level of toxins than at any time before.

That's all for now.

Eric

November 2005

Much of our e-mail comes from PALS who are improving or those who are not improving. I have a story about each one of those situations. First the story of no improvement. My standard answer for a no-improvement PALS is that they either have not done enough detox and/or they still have one or more toxins in their environment. Although I talk about an all-organic food diet in my book, the truth is that I had not been able to follow my own advice. Well, what can I say, except that everyone makes mistakes and I certainly have made one. For years now I have felt that I have been too slow in my improvement. After my San Diego visit to OHI (see September and October updates), I was talking about my experience with Dr. Kane. She suggested that my improvement at OHI was probably from something I was avoiding rather than something I was taking at OHI. I could not agree more. I'm now totally convinced that my improvement resulted more from avoiding toxins by eating organic food than the food itself. Also, I have read the book by Kevin Trudeau titled "Natural Cures "They" Don't Want You To Know About" You may want to read this book and if so you may order it by calling this number: (800) 709-6575. In his book, Kevin states that virtually every food product in the regular supermarket contains one or more toxic ingredients. I'm now convinced that is true. Remember, you probably cannot get well unless you avoid ALL toxins.

Here is a story about improvement and the need to be sure that you have eliminated every possible toxin from your environment. A Mr. A. Lee Vaughn from Renton, Washington sent me an e-mail about his problem. He said that when he went down to clean up the barn that he would develop a mild paralysis in his hands. Then, after returning to his house, the paralysis would go away after one or two hours. I sent him an e-mail suggesting that there must be something in his barn causing that; something toxic. I urged him to check his barn thoroughly for something toxic. He soon wrote back that he did that and discovered several cases of old mercury vapor street bulbs that were left by the previous owner who worked for the power company. I suggested that he have them removed and treated as a hazardous waste material. He has now done that and no longer has any problem cleaning out the barn and he is improving rapidly. If any of you had any doubt about how toxic mercury can be, that story should help you understand.

You might also be interested in the latest newsletter from DAMS. See my Regimen Outline for info on DAMS.

There is also a new web site about mercury that provides some very interesting facts.

http://www.mercola.com/article/mercury/mercury_elimination.htm

One more thing; it is apparent from reading our e-mail that not enough of you are following my Regimen Outline. When I finished writing my book, I realized that many of you would read the book and then not know what to do or what to do FIRST. That's why I made up the Regimen Outline and that's why it is in the exact order that I would do things if I were starting all over. Occasionally, I will add something to the Outline and/or edit it. I plan to do just that in the next few days, so I urge you to check it and look for the new revision. Also, if I were you I would print it and review it occasionally to make sure I was on track.

Here's to your good health,

Eric & Glenna

For the most current Updates which will continue, please review our web site:

http://www.ericiswinning.com/

REGIMEN OUTLINE (Revised 12-1-05)

TREATING A NEURO-DEGENERATIVE ILLNESS SUCH AS ALS

This outline is provided for two reasons; One is because many people read the book and don't know what to do first. Second, it lists all the main things you should consider doing.

These suggested treatments are in the order that I would do them if I were starting all over back in 1996.

I am not a healthcare professional and I'm not recommending any treatment for any individual. These treatments are all treatments that I have done and what I believe are responsible for my being alive today after fifteen years with ALS.

The only recommendation I make is that you take these suggestions to a healthcare professional and use this outline as a guide.

In the book I write about Phase One and Phase Two. I think there has been some confusion about that, so I'm changing it and I hope it will clarify what I mean. Actually, there are Type One treatments and Type Two treatments and there is Phase One and Phase Two. For example, Type One treatments are the primary treatments for Phase One. Some Type Two treatments are necessary for Phase One also. Type Two treatments are primary for Phase Two. If this sounds confusing, it may clear up with the following:

PHASE ONE OBJECTIVE – Stop the progress of ALS.

PHASE TWO OBJECTIVE – Restore the body to a more normal condition.

TYPE ONE TREATMENTS – You must treat the CAUSE and the cause is a toxin or toxins. They must be eliminated first. This includes any treatment to detoxify the body AND any treatment to avoid exposure to additional toxins. The primary treatments to detoxify are chelation, colon hydrotherapy, clay baths, etc. The primary treatments to avoid more toxins include eliminating dental mercury amalgams and eliminating toxic fungus, and mycoplasmas in your colon. Also, read all the Updates which include individual stories about eliminating toxins in your environment.

TYPE TWO TREATMENTS – THERE IS NO TYPE TWO TREATMENT THAT WILL CURE ALS, in my opinion. Type Two treatments are treatments that restore the body to its normal condition. Some Type Two treatments are included in Phase One as supplemental treatments but not primary. Type Two treatments include live cell therapy, supplements like Glyconutrients, and an all organic food diet, etc.

THE FOLLOWING OUTLINE OFFERS MORE INFORMATION ABOUT EACH TREATMENT. Although detox is your primary objective in Phase One, there are other things I would do before beginning detox.

1 – PREPARATION FOR DETOX

A – Establish a highly nutritious diet of many fresh vegetables, fresh fruit, nuts, AND ALL ORGANIC. Eat a minimum amount of meat or none. NO FISH. Eat much of your produce RAW. Some of this may be done with a juicer.

B – GLYCONUTRIENTS are probably the most important supplement of all.

They are required for cell-to-cell communication AND they help the body produce more of its own stem cells.

For more information on Glyconutrients or to place an order, call or send an e-mail to:

Mary Rose Ramirez
E-Mail: *PREC143@aol.com* (include "Glyconutrients" in the subject line)
Phone (307) 634-2444 (Home)
Phone (307) 221-0830 (Cell) Note: She lives in Wyoming, USA

NOTE

Glyconutrients can only be sold and shipped to the following countries:
United States, Canada, Korea, United Kingdom, Japan & New Zealand.

C – pH TEST – Check your pH level and you will probably find that you are acidic which is not good. You should have an alkaline pH of 7.0 or higher.

Generally speaking, a vegetarian diet plus Glyconutrients plus many minerals, including calcium, should do the trick.

Here is a number you can call for a pH test kit:

(800) 899-8349

D – TERRAMIN CLAY – A great way to raise your pH to a proper alkaline level is one teaspoon of Terramin clay in water twice a day. That works for me. This is an all natural clay with an abundance of minerals.

You can order Terramin clay from the following:

Maryanne Maldonado
http://www.i-amperfectlyhealthy.com/
phone (520) 219-2379

E – POMEGRANATE JUICE

Drink four ounces or more of ORGANIC pomegranate juice daily. For information read the December 2005 Update.

2 – SELECT A HEALTHCARE PROFESSIONAL – ACAM DOCTORS

I would urge you to divorce your present medical doctor unless he is open-minded to alternative treatments.

One way to locate a medical doctor in your area who does alternative treatments is to contact ACAM. The American College for Advancement in Medicine (ACAM) is a not-for-profit medical society dedicated to educating physicians and other healthcare professionals on latest findings and emerging procedures in preventive/nutritional medicine. Most of these doctors also do chelation treatments. However, not all of them have the same degree of chelation training. You still must be selective in your choice of a doctor.

ACAM represents more than 1,000 physicians in many countries. To find one in your area, you can contact them at the address below or look on their website:

The American College for Advancement in Medicine
23121 Verdugo Dr., Suite 204
Laguna Hills, CA 92653
Phone (949) 583-7666 or Toll Free Outside CA (800) 532-3688
http://www.acam.org//

3 – AVOID TOXINS

Eliminate exposure to all toxins in your environment; that includes toxins in your home, in your diet, in your water, amalgam removal, and toxins in your colon like fungus, bad bacteria, and mycoplasmas. Buy one or more air filters for your home. Install an adequate high-quality water filter. Eliminate all toxic items in your home such as household cleaners, personal care items like hair spray, and aluminum cooking pots. Eliminate all foods from your diet that may contain preservatives, MSG, Aspartame, or any other toxic ingredient. Better yet, eat only ORGANIC FOOD. Again, I would avoid all fresh water fish, all salt water fish and all other seafood. They contain mercury.

4 – AMALGAM REMOVAL

If I had any dental amalgams containing mercury, I would have them removed at once. Mercury is poison. It does not belong in your body. Additionally, I would remove any tooth that had a root canal procedure. You must find a dentist who is experienced in amalgam removal and will take all the necessary precautions during removal.

Some dentists may charge thousands of dollars for amalgam replacement. You don't have to pay that much. Check around. In 1998 my dentist charged me approximately $125 each to remove my two amalgam fillings and replace them with porcelain.

I would unquestionably call DAMS and request their INFORMATION KIT. The kit will include a wealth of information about dental work, specific instructions on amalgam removal, and a list of dentists in your area.

DAMS, Inc.
Phone (800) 311-6265

Here is another option. You may want to consider Hal Huggins, a dentist in Colorado, or a Huggins trained dentist. Huggins wrote the book "It's All In Your Head." Another PALS has some interesting comments about the Huggins procedure. See the May 2005 Update.

5 – LYME & MYCOPLASMAS

The tick bite causes Lyme disease by injection of toxins. Mycoplasmas in your colon cause toxins. As a part of your AVOIDING TOXINS you may want to consider testing for each of them. These are highly specialized tests. There is only one laboratory that I would rely on. They test for Lyme and mycoplasmas and much more. Here is their information:

Medical Diagnostic Laboratories
2439 Kuser Road
Hamilton, NJ 08690-3303
Phone (609) 570-1000
FAX (609) 570-1050
E-mail: *www.mdlab.com*

You may call them to request the necessary forms, but they must be completed by you AND the doctor.

6 – GET A HAIR ANALYSIS

This is a must. A hair analysis will provide you with much needed information about your system. It will tell you about toxic metals in your system. It will also tell you about minerals in your system.

Treatment should correspond to the analysis. Additionally, you can get future hair analyses and compare to chart your progress on eliminating metals from your system. If you do not have a hair analysis, you will be flying blind. A hair analysis may not be 100% accurate and it will not provide indication of ALL toxins. However, it's the only way you will have any clue about what's going on in your system.

Great Smokies Diagnostic Lab will only provide hair analysis kits for healthcare professionals. Ask your healthcare professional to order one for you from the following:

Great Smokies Diagnostic Lab
63 Zillicoa Ave.
Asheville, NC 28801
Phone (828) 253-0621

Here is an even better way to obtain a hair analysis

A doctor in Cincinnati, Ohio provides a hair analysis with a consultation by phone and/or e-mail to anyone worldwide. She is a nutritional consultant as well as an experienced hair analyst. Her full service, all by phone or e-mail, costs a little over $100 and I fully recommend it; it's worth every penny.

You may contact her by phone or e-mail to order the hair analysis kit.

Dr. Kathleen N. Akin, CCSP
Alternative & Wellness Center
Phone (513) 931-4300 or (888) 257-9608
Email: *qualitycarechiro@cinci.rr.com*
http://www.advancedfamilyhealth.com/

7 – COLON HYDROTHERAPY

This one is a must also. This treatment will help the body eliminate toxins. It should be done before, during and after amalgam removal and other detox treatments. It is very important that you clean out your colon with a hydrotherapy treatment before you begin a detox treatment. Detox will add more burden on your liver, kidneys, and colon. This is the first thing I did when I started my program and didn't know about anything else. Colon hydrotherapy along with an extreme diet plus many supplements was the primary cause of the reversal of my ALS condition. I think it would be a good idea to have several colon hydrotherapy treatments immediately. Additionally, I would have one very soon after amalgam removal and after any other detox treatment such as chelation or clay baths.

8 – WATER

I would drink at least eight glasses of pure water (not tap water) everyday. Most toxins are eliminated from your system through your bowels or your urinary system. Therefore, drinking a lot of pure water may be equally important to colon hydrotherapy. If you don't do this, the toxins will be recycled.

9 – COLLOIDAL SILVER – A NATURAL ANTIBIOTIC

You may want to consider adding colloidal silver to your diet. There are two reasons for this:

a. According to what I read, colloidal silver is an effective treatment for Lyme disease. Many PALS have been misdiagnosed with ALS when they really had Lyme. I have taken eight ounces of colloidal silver twice a day for a long time now without any bad side effects. If it were me, I would continue eight ounces twice a day for at least six months; that is, eight ounces of distilled water processed through the SilverGen generator (see below).

b. Colloidal silver is a natural antibiotic and has been known to effectively eliminate unwanted parasites from your colon. Most people, including 85% of all PALS, have excessive bad bacteria, fungus, and/or mycoplasmas in their colons.

If you are interested in making your own colloidal silver, there is a unit you can buy for about $200 US:

The SilverGen SG6 Automatic Colloid Generator
Phone (877) 745-8374 or (360) 732-5091
http://www.silvergen.com/

Probiotics

Most people old enough to have ALS also have bowel problems. Typically they have more bad bacteria than good bacteria in their colon. Although some people say "You are what you eat," that is not quite correct. You are what you properly digest. You must have a digestive system that works properly. You may consider doing two things. First, you may reduce the quantity of bad bacteria, etc. by taking a natural antibiotic like colloidal silver which we just discussed above. Then, second, you may take one or more probiotics to increase the quantity of the good bacteria in your colon. Pure natural yogurt and fermented foods like sauerkraut are natural probiotics. There are many more, but one I like is Probiotic Advantage by Dr. David Williams. You can call (800) 888-1415 to order.

Note: You may take colloidal silver and probiotics at the same time according to what I read. Colloidal silver only kills the bad bacteria and not the good. Prescription antibiotic drugs kill all bacteria and should be avoided.

10 – DETOXIFYING YOUR BODY

The number one goal is the elimination of heavy metals and other toxins which have accumulated in your body over the years. Detox is not listed first in this outline only because there are other things that I would do before undertaking any detox treatment.

Originally, I thought that chelation was the very best way to detox for mercury and other heavy metals. Then I learned about Bentonite clay. DMPS chelation by IV is a proven way to eliminate mercury from your body. However, Bentonite clay may be more suitable for someone who has advanced symptoms and/or is too frail. The clay baths can be regulated by the amount of clay in the bath, length of time soaking, and the frequency of bathing. Additionally, the clay baths can be done in your home and they are relatively inexpensive.

If it were me, I would probably do both but not at the same time. I might do clay baths for a while and then switch to chelation. You may want to have a urine analysis immediately following any detox treatment so that you will have some indication of what the treatment is pulling out of your system.

It is possible that different methods of detoxification may remove toxins from different parts of the body. Therefore, it might be wise to do two or more different TYPES of detox treatments.

Number of Treatments

I'm often asked the question "How many detox treatments should I have?" My answer is "All that you need to make your body as pure and pristine as possible." That may take ten or twenty chelation treatments for one person, or forty or fifty for another person. The same answer applies to chelation, clay baths or any other detox treatment. Again, this is why you need a periodic hair analysis to chart your progress.

Chelation

You should locate an ACAM doctor in your area who does IV chelation. See the previous discussion about ACAM doctors.

LL's Magnetic Clay

LL's Magnetic Clay provides a kit made of Bentonite clay plus additives for detoxification of heavy metals. There are various kits for detox of different heavy metals. Specific instructions are included in the kit. You add the clay (powder) to your bath water and soak your entire body in it, or you can just do a foot bath as I do. This may sound a little mysterious but I know that it works. For more information on this, visit the web site below.

I've only had experience with clay from LL's Magnetic Clay. Your hair analysis will provide the information for you to decide which kit to use. If you're still unsure, I would order two different clay kits; one for general detox and one for mercury detox. You might want to alternate them.

For general health information, you may visit this web site

http://www.evenbetternow.com/

For a complete overview of LL's Magnetic Clay and how it works, go to

http://www.evenbetterhealth.com/magnetic-clay.html

For more specific information on LL's Magnetic Clay and ALS, go to

http://www.als-options.com/detoxification-therapy.html

To order by phone call (Evenbetternow, LLC) Toll-Free at (877) 562-6039. Questions and International Orders call (520) 877-2637

Dr. Patricia Kane

Dr. Kane has had great success treating ALS patients with her treatment protocol which is different from anything else in this outline. I followed her protocol for about three months and I know that it works. It is not a "do-it- yourself" program, so you must contact her for more information. It is not inexpensive, but if you have a few dollars to spare, you might contact her and I do recommend her program. She is wonderful to work with.

If any of you are interested in more information about Dr. Kane's protocol, you may contact her office:

Haverford Wellness Center
Dr. Domenick Braccia
Dr. Patricia Kane
2010 West Chester Pike
Suite 310
Havertown, PA 19083

Phone: (610) 924-0600
Fax: (610) 924-0600
http://www.haverfordwellness.com/

There is one part of her protocol that you could do yourself and that I know has helped me. She recommends a product called E-Lyte. This product contains electrolytes and may be added to your drinking water. It works.

Bionic Cleansing

It may sound crazy, but it works. You put your feet in a tub of water with an electrical instrument and it draws toxins out of your body through your feet. You know it is working because after a few minutes the water will change color in accordance with the type of toxin being eliminated.

To locate a doctor that has this equipment and is trained in its use, call Energy Balance Resources shown under Laser Treatment of Phase Two of this outline.

Optimum Health Institute

Glenna and I went to this clinic for one week and had amazing results. It is another one that is not inexpensive, but what you learn and the experience is well worth it. You stay there for one, two or three weeks. They feed you only RAW food that is ALL ORGANIC. This is where I learned the true value of an all-organic diet. Avoiding MSG and preservatives is just not enough. For more information about our experience at this clinic, please read the Updates of September, October and November 2005.

Here is their information:

Optimum Health Institute
San Diego, California
Phone (619) 464-3346 or (800) 993-4325
Web site: *http://www.optimumhealth.org/*

They also have another clinic in Texas.

Phase One Conclusion

If for any reason you are unable to do most of the above, here is the minimum that I would do.

    a. Detoxify
    b. Avoid toxins
    c. Eat only organic food
    d. Correct your pH to alkaline
    e. Eliminate all amalgam dental fillings
    f. Take Glyconutrients

The above are all the Phase One treatments I would do plus the live cell therapy discussed under Phase Two below.

PHASE TWO

RESTORING THE BODY

The purpose of Phase Two is to restore your body to a more normal condition. The primary treatments are all Type Two treatments to restore. Exactly when you should start Phase Two treatments is an unknown. Some Phase One treatments such an organic diet and Glyconutrients may be continued in Phase Two. The following treatments may be started anytime, but they may not be as effective as you might hope for until after you have done more of the Type One treatments. For example; the live cell therapy which will be discussed next, may not be effective if you begin it too soon. The toxins in your body may destroy the new live cells faster than you can take them and they are not cheap. You must decide when.

1 – LIVE CELL THERAPY

You have heard of stem cell therapy and this is not exactly the same. Generally speaking, all types of cell transplant therapy are basically the same. Cell therapy is probably one of the greatest new treatments in many years. The live cell therapy I have been following is possibly the most effective for the cost. Based on my experience, this really is amazing. Remember, however, this is a Type Two treatment. Since it does not treat the cause of any health problem, it is doomed to failure unless you eliminate the cause of your health problem first or at the same time.

The supplies for the live cell therapy that I'm taking and more information is available on the following web site:

http://www.als-options.com/ or
http://www.als-options.com/live-cell-therapy.html

To order by phone call (Evenbetternow, LLC) Toll-Free at (877) 562-6039. Questions and International Orders call (520) 877-2637.

They offer four items: three are liquid and one is a capsule. I am only taking two of the liquids which are BRAIN CELLS and LIVER CELLS and this works fine for me. I take one liver dose in the morning and one brain dose in the evening before my meal. This is not inexpensive but about 1% of the cost for the China stem cell treatment. Please do not overlook this treatment because of the expense. If you cannot afford to do what I'm doing, then take only the brain cell treatment and/or take it less often BUT TAKE IT. It is simply too good to ignore entirely. Since I switched to an all-organic diet AND began this therapy, I have had more improvement in a short time than in anytime previously.

If you do the above live cell therapy, you may not need any of the following treatments. However, they are included for your consideration anyway.

2 – VITAMIN B-1 TREATMENT

There was a medical doctor right here in California who developed an apparently successful treatment for ALS and MS patients. This was a few decades ago, and he is dead now. One of his patients lived more than thirty years after the treatment.

The treatment involved an abundance of supplements not too different from all those in my book. However, two items were very different:

    a. 400 mg of Vitamin B-1 INJECTIONS daily. Note: I've read that it is good for the nervous system and helps the body detoxify.
    b. Injections of liver extract.

I am currently doing injections of 200 mg of B-1 daily and 200 mg B-1 orally. Part of the live cell therapy that I'm taking includes live liver cells.

3 – VITAMIN/MINERAL IV

The vitamin/mineral plus glutathione IV I have been doing now for several years. This IV treatment is done in conjunction with chelation. However, you may want to continue this treatment, as I have, for Phase Two.

4 – HUMAN GROWTH HORMONE

I have now been taking a daily shot of HGH for a year and a half. It is a little expensive, but I know it works for me. It comes in many forms but I selected a throw-away syringe. It has no preservatives because you mix it in the syringe just before you apply it. The needle is so fine that most of the time I don't even feel it. My wife, who would never give me a regular shot of anything, gives me this shot everyday with no problem. You can only obtain this with a prescription from your MD.

5 – STARBUCKS

Now you're going to laugh when I tell you this one. However, I am dead serious. I truly believe that the drink that I buy at Starbucks everyday is helping me. They make a Chai Tea latte with soy milk. Chai Tea is a black tea which has antioxidants in it. Additionally, Starbucks adds many spices such as ginger, cinnamon, etc. Now I have no idea whether it is the tea, the spices, or the soy milk, but I don't care. I do not suggest this for anyone, but I know it has helped me.

6 – LASER TREATMENT

This is simply a laser beam that the doctor will shine on your body and move around. I would call it a stimulator. It apparently stimulates your nerves, your muscles, your brain and your body organs. For that reason, it is a little bit of Phase One and Phase Two. When it stimulates your organs, it may be helping your body to eliminate toxins. My doctor does arm muscle testing to evaluate the effect of the laser treatment. Now I know first hand by the muscle testing that this one works.

You may be able to locate a doctor in your area who has this equipment by calling the manufacturer:

Energy Balance Resources
Phone (866) 522-5262
http://www.4ebr.com/

7 – POSITIVE MENTAL ATTITUDE

Last but not least, you must remember PMA and prayer. Additionally, you must take charge of your own health care. Do not relinquish this to any other single person. Again, all the above treatments are only the more important ones. This outline is just to give you the highlights of what one can do for ALS or any of the other forty or more neuro-degenerative ailments.

Glenna and I wish you well.

Eric Edney

NO ONE EVER ACCOMPLISHED
ANYTHING WORTHWHILE WITHOUT PMA
(POSITIVE MENTAL ATTITUDE)
FIRST PMA – THEN SUCCESS

This Regimen Outline may change occasionally. The latest revision will be posted on our web site:

http://www.ericiswinning.com/

Printed in the United States
82196LV00002B/117